MENIERE MAN
IN THE HIMALAYAS

LOW SALT CURRIES

Low Salt Cooking In The Kitchens Of India

PAGE ADDIE PRESS
GREAT BRITAIN AND AUSTRALIA

Copyright

CONTENTS

I

Even in the poorest households,
Indians look forward to sharing a meal with guests.
There is a saying in India,
"If a crow sits on your window sill in the early morning
and caws away - you are sure to have visitors".

There is also an ancient Sanskrit saying

'The Guest is your God'

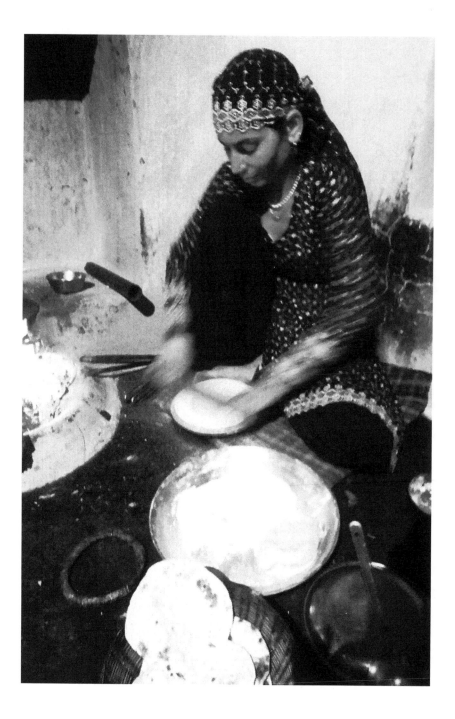

THE JOURNEY
OF LOW SALT COOKING
IN THE KITCHENS OF INDIA

Being here in the vast Indian subcontinent and eating low salt has certainly been a challenge. This project came about by necessity. It all started on the first night I arrived in New Delhi. I was invited to join friends for dinner at a famous colonial restaurant in Connaught Place. I ordered the most popular dish on the menu since 1938, the Rhaj vindaloo, with pappadums. It was delicious, yet so heavily salted I couldn't finish it.

Lunch the next day at the hotel restaurant was the same story. The spices of the chicken cooked in the Tandor oven were wonderfully blended, but it seemed like the top had come off the salt shaker. After that I avoided ordering curries. Yet this was India! The food is legendary. I hadn't come here to eat pizza.

During my three days in Delhi, I had been returning to the same restaurant and only eating garlic naan and rice. This time the owner, Anju Japoor, asked me why I never ordered her curries. I explained that I couldn't eat salted food due to a medical condition. She was very empathetic and told me that her father had two bypass heart surgeries. She looked at me and asked my age. When I told her, she put her hand over her heart, closed her eyes and drew a deep breath. "You are the same age as my father, I miss him." She placed her hand on my arm and invited me into her kitchen. "Wash your hands," she said. Then she pulled down a wooden board, handed me a sharp knife, and asked me to chop four purple onions, a large head of garlic, a knuckle size piece of ginger root, and a bunch of green coriander (while I was at it).

That afternoon, Anju showed me how to cook her famous (in all of India) Paneer Tika Masala, using no salt. The next evening we made her Lamb Biryani without salt or red chillies. She watched me eat it and quizzed me on the taste. I assured her the dish was truly memorable. It was creamy, delicious and aromatic. She dipped her spoon into the rich sauce, patted me on the arm and said, "This is a good idea, this no salt." From then on she called me "Papa."

In Himachal Pradesh, I was invited into the home of a local family to eat dinner. Naan toasted over the open fire. Dahl and rice served up on large metal plates. It was a wonderful experience to share traditional food with a local family. The next night I was invited again. This time, I had to explain that I couldn't eat salt. Thoughtfully they prepared my portion of the dinner separately, without adding salt. However, just removing a flavor condiment like salt made the food on the plate very bland. When you don't add salt, it's important to add the right spices and herbs for taste.

Complimentary condiments are essential in all cooking, especially in curries. Creating delicious low salt Indian curries in this book, can be as subtle as listening to the pop and sizzle of cumin seeds as you add them at the perfect temperature. Spices "speak" their own language.

While traveling through India, I made friends with local chefs and Indian foodies, who shared their favorite recipes with me. The important point we all agreed on was this. Yes, you can cook curries without picking up the salt shaker. But, to create a truly memorable taste experience without salt, curries require subtle ingredient adjustments; to the dry spices, the masala paste, and the herbs. Indian cooking is about getting the balance of all the ingredients for authentic taste and flavor. This is what cooking *Low Salt Curries* is all about.

Writing this book about curries, I discovered that curries are not just about culinary taste but about promoting good health as well. From cinnamon to cardamom, mint to coriander - spices and herbs have powerful health giving benefits. Knowing this has certainly deepened my love of Indian curries. So for those who love curries and must avoid salt, here are authentic *low salt* curry recipes, as cooked with gracious open hearted friends in the kitchens' of India.

THE HEALTH BENEFITS OF CURRIES

Cooking curries with spices like turmeric, cumin, cinnamon and ginger is a natural way to enhance overall body health. Spices and herbs not only add culinary flavor but have powerful medicinal values.

India is the land of spices. Ayurvedic, the 5000 year old medical practice of India, encompasses the healing of body, mind and spirit through the use of spices and herbs in the diet. They have known for centuries that food and diet can have a profound effect on health. For example, 1 teaspoon of paprika has 16% of the bodies daily requirement of vitamin A, in the form of beta carotene. Spices also contain potent antioxidants which protect against disease.

During the Roman Empire, spices were more valuable than gold. Europe had salt but wanted more flavor and taste. Trade routes opened between Rome and India. Spice traders brought peppercorns, cinnamon, cardamon, nutmeg and a myriad of other precious spices to the tables of Europe.

During that era of history, the benefits of spices were common knowledge. Spices could add taste and zest to meals, promote good health, slow down the aging process, help with weight loss, fight against disease and banish pain. Spices were valuable. Rare, precious and treasured. One ounce of saffron was worth more than a pound of gold.

16

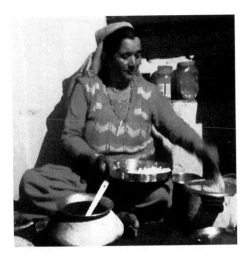

CURRY BASICS

In Indian cooking, a blend of fragrant spices in dry or paste form is known as a masala. Masala is the Hindi word for 'spice mixture'. Spices vary according to the recipe and region. Variations of masala for the same recipe exist with its own unique spice blend and specific use. You can add or subtract spices and vary the amount to please you and your family's palate. This is the way curry recipes have evolved since antiquity.

Curries are often in the form of a yogurt, cream or coconut based sauce made with a masala mixture of cumin, cinnamon, turmeric and many other aromatic spices. Masala can been found by name in restaurants here and the spicy blends are used to flavor meals in home kitchens. For example Chicken Tika Masala is made with masala paste in a creamy tomato based orange colored sauce.

Often spices for masala are fried (roasted) for a richer flavor before being made into a paste or powder. You can use a clean nut mill for grinding, a food processor, blender or a mortar and pestle. When you see masala paste in the following recipes in this book, first make the masala fresh and set aside. Then prepare the rest of the curry.

For pungent curry recipes, the powder called *garam masala* may be an additional seasoning favorite. Translated as "spicy mixture" it is a ready made blend of traditional Indian spices. *Garam masala* contains health benefits of black pepper, cardamon, cinnamon, cloves and other spices in the blend. You buy *garam masala powder*, (along with other spices found in the recipes), in supermarkets, specialty food stores and delicatessens.

The trick with spices is to buy small quantities, store them in glass jars, away from heat and light. Spices will lose their potency after a while, so keep your spices up to date. That dented green tin of Bombay curry powder, bought ten years ago, won't cut the mustard! Replace spices regularly. Be sure to use fresh ingredients when you cook Indian food.

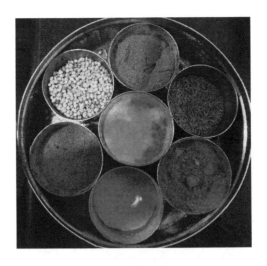

GO JUNGLEE

Once you understand the basics of Indian cooking, you can go junglee, which is a Hindi saying meaning wild or crazy. Junglee is not about adding salt or chillies for flavor and heat, but being creative with fresh herbs and exotic spices. A pinch more of cumin seeds. An extra grind of black pepper. Another cardamon pod or two.

The very nature of this great Indian subcontinent cuisine is that the recipes have been adapted by cooks, royal chefs and local families for centuries to suit their tastes. So here's to adding spice to your life and doing a bit of *low salt* junglee, with Meniere Man and friends in the Himalayas.

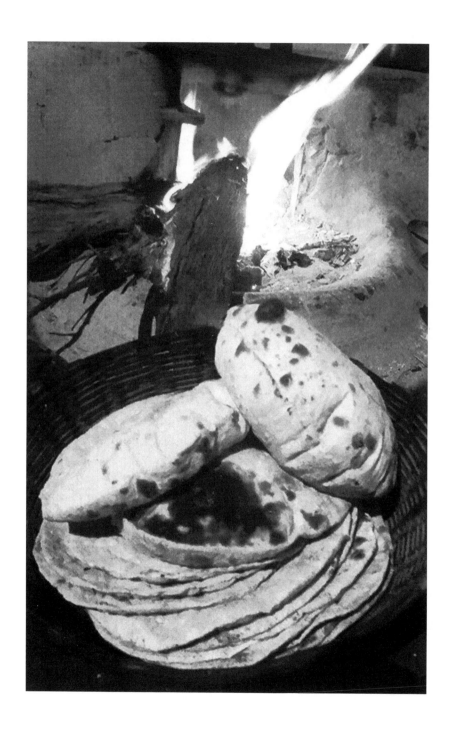

HIMACHAL PRADESH

While the local people of Himachal Pradesh like very spicy food, the day to day food is northern Indian style, consisting of dal (a preparation of pulses, dried lentils, peas or beans) and rice or roti (wheat based flat bread). Most often dal is served as a stew on the plate, which you mop up with flat bread and rice. Dal is comparable to meat in protein value, making it a valuable fat free carbohydrate.

MIXED VEGETABLE PAKORA

Mixed vegetable pakora is a hot crispy snack.
Easy and quick to make.

Serves 6 - 8

Cooking time: 30 minutes

Ingredients

250g chick pea flour

50g plain unbleached flour

1 tsp baking powder

1 tsp garam masala

1 tsp cumin

1 tsp turmeric powder

1 tsp garam masala

1 tsp fresh squeezed lemon juice

3 - 3 1/2 cups of any of the following vegetables

potatoes, peeled, finely sliced

red or brown onions, cut in thin rings

cauliflower, cut into small florets

carrots, peeled, cut in 1 cm pieces

French beans, cut in 1 cm pieces

cabbage, finely shredded

green peas, shelled (or frozen)

Method

Place flours, baking powder together with spices in a mixing bowl. Add lemon juice and enough water to make a smooth batter. Set aside for 10 minutes. Add all remaining ingredients to the batter, except the sunflower oil. Mix well, coating all the vegetables. Heat oil in a frying pan. Do not leave pan unattended. When oil is hot, place 1 tablespoon of the batter into the hot oil. Use a slotted spoon. Fry in small batches for 5-6 minutes until the vegetables are cooked and golden brown. Drain on kitchen paper. Serve immediately.

PALAK PANEER
Paneer cooked in smooth spinach tomato curry.

Serves: 6
Cooking time: 45 minutes

Ingredients

250g fresh paneer (see recipe for paneer) cubed and lightly fried
3 large bunches of English or baby spinach, washed (discard stems)

1-2 tsp unsalted butter

1 tsp cumin seeds

2 medium onions, chopped then boiled in a little water and drained.

1 tsp ginger paste

1 tsp garlic paste

1 tbsp coriander powder

2 large tomatoes (blanched in hot water, peeled)

1 cup water (use spinach cooking water)

1 tsp garam masala

1 tbsp (or more) cream, as garnish

Method

Chop spinach. Blanch spinach in a pan with 1 cup boiling water. Drain. Save cooking water. Set aside. Melt butter in a heavy bottomed pan. Add cumin seeds. Heat until you hear them "pop". Add garlic and ginger paste. Fry 4 minutes. Blend tomatoes with onions. Add to frying pan. Fry until brown taking care not to burn. Add coriander powder. Add spinach. Cook 3 minutes. Add paneer cubes. Add the water that spinach was blanched in, as required. Cook on medium heat for 10 minutes. Add garam masala. Mix together well. Reduce heat. Cook 3 minutes. Run a swirl of pouring cream in a circular pattern to garnish the finished dish. Serve hot with steamed rice or chapattis.

VEGETABLE KORMA
A rich yellow creamy vegetable curry with a
hint of sweet cashew nuts.

Serves: 6 - 8
Cooking time: 30 minutes

Ingredients

2 large brown onions, diced

3 large tomatoes, boiled, skinned, chopped

1 cm fresh ginger root, finely chopped

1 head garlic, peeled and finely chopped

2 large potatoes, peeled, thinly sliced

4 carrots, peeled, diced

1/2 cauliflower, cut in small florets

1 cup pumpkin, cut in small cubes

3 tbsp unsalted cashew nuts, blended

4 large tomatoes, boiled and skinned

1 cup peas, fresh (or frozen)

1 cup fresh cream (or plain yogurt)

3 cardamom pods, crushed

2 tsp coriander

1 tsp turmeric

1 tsp garam masala

sunflower oil

Method

Boil potatoes, carrots, peas, pumpkin, and cauliflower until tender. Boil tomatoes and onion in 1/2 cup water. Remove skin on tomatoes. Blend onions and tomatoes together to make a tomato paste. Heat 1 tbsp of oil in a large pan. Cook onion and spices until aromatic. Add garlic and ginger. Cook 2 minutes. Add vegetables and tomato/onion paste. Cook on low heat 5-10 minutes. Remove from heat. Stir in yogurt/or cream. Heat gently. Take off heat. Add chopped fresh coriander leaves.
Serve hot with basmati rice or naan bread.

MALI KOFTA

Melt in the mouth dumplings immersed in a creamy, mild red curry sauce.

Serves: 4 - 6
Cooking time: 20 minutes

Ingredients

makes 10 koftas
2 large potatoes, boiled, mashed
1/2 cup carrots, chopped

1/2 cup French beans, cut in 1 cm pieces

1/2 cup peas, fresh, shelled (or frozen)

1/2 cup cauliflower, broken into small florets

1/2 cup fresh paneer, crumbled

2 tsp coriander

1 tsp cumin

2 tbsp cashew nuts

2 tbsp raisins

2 tbsp coriander leaves, chopped

1 tsp corn flour

corn flour for rolling koftas

sunflower oil

Masala Paste

Ingredients

1 large brown onion

fresh ginger, 2cm finely chopped

one head garlic, peeled and chopped

3 large tomatoes, boiled and skinned

1 tsp turmeric powder

1 tsp cumin seeds

2 tsp coriander powder

1/4 cup pouring cream

1 tbsp cashew nuts, coarsely chopped

1 tsp garam masala

pistachio nuts, shelled
raisins
sunflower oil

Method

Boil vegetables for 10 minutes until tender. Drain.
Save potato water. Grate the paneer. Mix grated
paneer with mashed potatoes, cooked vegetables,
coriander, cumin, coriander leaves, nuts and 1 tsp
corn flour. Break off a small piece and flatten. Place
a few raisins and pistachio nuts, into dough, before
shaping each into a cylinder. Roll in corn flour. Set
aside. Heat fry pan with oil. Fry koftas in small batches
until golden brown. Remove with slotted spoon and
place to drain on kitchen towels while you make the
sauce.

Masala Sauce

Method

Heat 1 tbsp oil in a pan. Fry onions until golden brown,
taking care not to burn. Add garlic and ginger. Saute
for 3 minutes. Add tomatoes, turmeric, coriander, and
cumin. Cook for 2 minutes. Add 2 tbsp water if too dry.
Cool. When cool blend to a smooth paste.
Heat pan with 1 tsp oil. Add cumin seeds and cook

until they "pop". Add blended paste. Add 1 cup of water, cream and cashew nut powder. Bring to the boil. Turn heat down to low. Add koftas to sauce. To serve, place in serving dish. Add a swirl of fresh cream to garnish. Sprinkle with finely chopped coriander leaves. Serve hot with chapatti or naan.

PANEER BUTTER MASALA
Soft paneer in a creamy tomato gravy.

Serves: 6
Cooking time: 45 minutes

Ingredients

200 -250g paneer, cubed
2 tbsp cashew nuts, 2 tbsp poppy seeds, 2 tbsp melon seeds, blended in a little water to a paste
5 medium tomatoes, boiled lightly, skinned and blended
1cm piece fresh ginger, peeled, finely chopped
5 cloves garlic, peeled, finely chopped
sunflower oil
2 tbsp butter

1 tsp fenugreek

2 bay leaves

1 tbsp fresh mint leaves (stalks removed)

1 tsp garam masala

1 1/2 cups water

fresh coriander leaves for garnish

sugar to taste

Method

Blend garlic and ginger together with a 1 tsp of water. Heat 1 tbsp of sunflower oil and butter in a large frying pan. Add bay leaves and fry 10 seconds. Add ginger and garlic puree. Fry for 1 minute. Add tomato puree. Add cashew paste. Stir. Add water. Simmer on low heat. Add paneer. Cook 2-3 minutes until soft. Don't overcook, or paneer will become tough. Add crushed mint leaves, fenugreek and garam masala. Add water to thin. Add cream if you want a richer taste. Serve hot. Garnish with coriander leaves. Serve with plain naan bread, garlic naan or steamed rice.

SHAHI PANEER
A rich, aromatic Mughlai curry.

Serves 6

Cooking time: 40 minutes

Ingredients

250g paneer

1 cup onion stock

1/2 cup full fat plain yogurt

2 tbsp pouring cream (optional)

1 tsp cardamom powder

1/4 tsp saffron powder

1 tsp coriander powder

1 tsp turmeric powder

1 tsp garam masala powder

Onion Paste

Ingredients

2 medium onions, chopped

5 cloves garlic, peeled

1 cm fresh ginger, peeled and finely chopped

2 tbsp unsalted cashew nuts

1 tbsp dried melon seeds (without skin)

1 tbsp almonds

Method

Place onions, ginger, garlic, cashews, almonds and melon seeds in a large saucepan. Add 1 cup cold water. Simmer 10 minutes until onions are soft. Strain onions. Set onion stock aside. Place onion/ spice mixture into a blender. Add 2 tsp of onion stock. Blend well.

Aromatic Mix

Ingredients

1 bay leaf
3 cloves
3 green cardamom pods, crushed
2 black cardamom pods, crushed
1 cm cinnamon stick
1 tsp poppy seeds
3 tbsp butter or 3 tbsp sunflower oil

Method

Heat 3 tablespoons of sunflower oil (or 3 tbsp butter) in a frying pan. Fry the aromatic mix. Add blended onion paste. Saute. Add dry spice powders. Add yogurt and onion stock, water and 1/4 tsp sugar. Simmer on low heat for 10 minutes. Add cardamom

powder and saffron. Stir in the paneer. Add cream.
Simmer 2 minutes until the paneer is soft. Garnish with
chopped coriander leaves. Serve with naan bread,
rotis or jeera rice.

NAVRATAN KORMA

This royal dish is named after the Navratan-
the nine jewels of the great Mugal emperor
Akbar.

Serves: 6
Cooking time: 25 minutes

Ingredients

2 carrots, cut into small cubes
2 medium potatoes, cut into small cubes
1/4 - 1/2 cauliflower, broken into florets
12 French beans, sliced into 1 cm pieces
4 onions, sliced
1/2 head garlic, peeled, chopped finely
2 cm fresh ginger, peeled, finely chopped
1/2 cup green peas, shelled or frozen
1/2 cup raw cashew nuts
sunflower oil
30g melon seeds, black husk removed

1 tsp poppy seeds

6 green cardamom pods

2 cloves

4 black peppercorns

2 cm cinnamon sticks

2 cm fresh ginger, peeled, chopped finely

100 - 150g paneer, cut in cubes

1/2 cup plain yogurt

1/2 cup light pouring cream

1 tbsp raisins

Method

Heat 2 tsp of oil in a pan. Add fresh paneer. Fry until golden take care not to overcook. Paneer should be soft. Cook onions in 1/2 cup of water. Blend to a paste and set aside.

Wash and chop vegetables. Simmer vegetables in 3 cups unsalted boiling water until tender. Drain.

Soak cashew nuts in warm water for 10 minutes. Place in blender. Blend with melon and poppy seeds to a smooth paste.

Heat oil in a frying pan. Add cinnamon, cardamoms, peppercorns and cloves until aromatic. Add onion paste. Cook 5 minutes. Add ginger-garlic paste. Add yogurt. Stir over low heat. Add cashew nut paste. Cook 5 minutes.

Add boiled vegetables. Cook 3 minutes. Add 1/2 cup

water. Add paneer. Cook 1 minute. Swirl fresh cream through as a garnish.

Decorate with chopped cashews, pistachios or raisins.

AROMATIC POTATOES WITH CUMIN SEEDS

The humble inexpensive potato, meets exotic Indian herbs and spices.

Serves: 6

Cooking time: 20 minutes

Ingredients

5 medium potatoes, cut into small cubes, boiled

1 tbsp sunflower oil

2 tsp cumin seeds

1 tbsp fresh ginger, thinly sliced

2 tsp coriander seeds

1 tsp turmeric

2 tbsp coriander leaves, chopped

Method

Heat oil in a frying pan. Add cumin seeds and they will "pop". Add ginger.

Cook for 3 minutes. Reduce heat. Add remaining spices. Stir for 30 seconds. Add potatoes and mix well. Fry 5 minutes. Remove from heat. Place in serving dish. Add fresh coriander. Mix well. Serve hot.

MUSHROOM MATAR MASALA
Mushrooms sauteed with onions and spices.

Serves: 6
Cooking time: 30 minutes

Ingredients

4 green cardamom pods

2 cm cinnamon stick

3 medium onions, peeled and finely chopped

2 cm fresh garlic, finely chopped and blended

5 cloves garlic, peeled and blended

4 medium tomatoes, skinned and chopped

1 tsp turmeric

1 tbsp coriander powder

1 tsp garam masala

1/2 cup cashew nuts, blended with 1 cup water into a paste

2 cups green peas, shelled (or use frozen)
200g mushrooms, washed, cut into medium pieces
4 tbsp sunflower oil

Method

Heat oil in a fry pan. Saute cardamom pods, cinnamon and onions until brown. Add ginger paste. Add garlic paste. Cook 30 seconds. Add tomatoes. Add coriander powder, turmeric and garam masala. Cook 3 minutes. Add cashew paste. Add 1 cup water. Bring to boil. Add peas and mushrooms. Cook until peas are cooked. Serve hot with rice or rotis.

DUM ALOO

Baby potatoes in a creamy, smooth sauce.

excellent

Serves: 6
Cooking time: 40 minutes

Ingredients

12 baby potatoes halved or 6 medium potatoes cut in 1/8ths
12 cashew nuts
1 large onion, chopped

2 cm fresh ginger, peeled and finely chopped

3 cloves garlic, peeled and finely chopped

2 medium tomatoes, blended

4 green cardamom pods

2 cm cinnamon stick

1 tsp fennel powder

1 tsp garam masala

1 tsp turmeric

1 tsp coriander powder

3 tbsp plain yogurt

2 tbsp coriander leaves, chopped (garnish)

1 tsp. five spice instead of individual ground spices.

Method

Wash potatoes, wipe dry on kitchen paper. Heat oil in a shallow frying pan. Add potatoes. Cook until browned and tender. Remove from pan and drain. Set aside. Blend cashew nuts with 1 tbsp water to make a paste. Set aside. Blend onion, ginger and garlic together. Heat oil. Add cardamom and cinnamon until aromatic. Add garlic, ginger and onion paste. Brown the paste well. Add tomato puree and stir. Cook 4 minutes. Add spice powders. Fry until the oil separates from the mixture. Add cashew nut paste. Stir and fry until the oil leaves the ingredients and bubbles at the side of the pan. Add 3 cups water. Stir well. Bring curry to a boil. Add fried potatoes. Simmer until thickens. Add yogurt. Serve hot with rotis, rice or naan bread.

GAJAR MATER
A colorful, mildly spiced, carrot and pea curry.

Serves: 4
Cooking time: 30 minutes

Ingredients

1 tsp cumin seeds
2 cm fresh ginger, peeled and grated
1 tsp garam masala
5 medium carrots, peeled, chopped
1 cup peas, fresh shelled (or frozen)
sunflower oil
1/2 cup water
chopped coriander leaves (garnish)

Method

Heat oil in a frying pan. Add cumin seeds and fry until they "pop". Add ginger. Add garam masala. Fry for 1 minute. Add carrots and peas. Saute for 4 minutes. Add 1/2 cup water. Stir. Cover pan with a lid and reduce heat to low. Simmer, stirring occasionally. When vegetables are cooked, place in serving bowl. Garnish with coriander leaves. Serve hot.

MATAR PANEER

A simple north Indian recipe for a creamy tomato based curry.

Serves: 6

Cooking time: 20 minutes

Ingredients

250g fresh paneer

1 cup peas, fresh (or frozen)

2 cups water

1 tsp turmeric

1 tsp garam masala powder

1 tsp coriander powder

2 tbsp butter

coriander leaves (garnish)

sugar as needed

Masala Paste

Ingredients

4 medium tomatoes, skinned and chopped

2 medium onions, chopped

1 cm fresh ginger, peeled and chopped

4 cloves garlic, peeled and chopped

1 tbsp coriander leaves, chopped

5 cashew nuts, chopped

Blend aromatic paste ingredients together to make a smooth paste. Set aside.

Method

Cook peas in boiling water. Drain. Heat butter in a pan. Add cumin seeds and fry until they "pop". Add the masala paste to the pan. Fry for 5-7 minutes or until the oil separates from the paste. Add dry spices. Add peas. Stir. Add a little water if too thick. Add cubes of paneer. Cook. Take care not to overcook the paneer. Garnish with coriander leaves. Serve hot with naan or plain rice.

DAL MAKHANI

This rich and hearty dish of red kidney beans and lentils is full of fiber and protein.

Serves: 6

Cooking time: 30 minutes

Ingredients

3/4 cup whole black lentils (dal)

1 tsp cumin seeds

1 tbsp fresh ginger, peeled and finely chopped

4 cloves garlic, peeled and finely chopped

4 large tomatoes, stewed in a little water, skinned and pureed

2 tbsp pouring cream

2 tsp pouring cream (for garnish)

2 tsp mint, washed (stalks removed) finely chopped

1/2 tsp garam masala

1 tbsp butter

Method

Wash dal. Soak in hot water for 30 minutes. Discard water. Place dal in a pan and add 3 cups water. Bring to boil. Cover and simmer for approximately 30 minutes, until soft.

Soak mint in hot water for 10 minutes.

When dal is cooked, mash until soft and creamy.
Add some water if necessary. Heat butter in a heavy
bottomed saucepan. Add cumin seeds. Stir until they
"pop". Add garlic. Brown. Add 1 cup tomato puree. Add
ginger. Cook on medium heat for 8 minutes. Add a
little water if needed.
Turn heat to low. Add dal. Stir. Add cream. Cover pan.
Simmer 10 minutes, stir every 2 minutes until creamy.
Add mint and soaking water. Cook 5 minutes on low
heat. Stirring. Add garam masala. Cook 3 minutes.
Remove from heat. Garnish with a swirl of cream or
plain yogurt. Serve hot with rice, rotis or naan bread.
Serve with finely chopped red onions.

CHANA DAL

Tasty aromatic vegetarian split pea curry.
High in protein.

Serves: 6
Cooking time: 40 minutes

Ingredients

250g chana dal (yellow dried split peas), rinsed
1 liter water
3 tbsp sunflower oil
1 tbsp cumin seeds
1 medium onion, chopped
2 cm fresh ginger, peeled and cut in thin strips
4 cloves garlic, peeled and left whole
4 large tomatoes
1 tsp turmeric
1 tsp garam masala
2 tsp coriander powder
ground black pepper
fresh coriander leaves
pouring cream

Method

Take a large pan. Add lentil and 800 mls water. Stir.
Bring to boil. Cover with lid. Simmer on low heat for
40 minutes, stirring occasionally. Add more water if
needed. Remove from heat when lentils are cooked.
Whisk lentils make a puree. Cool.

Heat oil in a frying pan. Add cumin. Stir until cumin
seeds "pop". Add onion and ginger. Fry 5 minutes. Set
aside. Blend garlic and tomatoes in a food processor.
Add puree to frying pan. Add spices and 100 mls
water. Simmer over medium heat 10 minutes, or
until the oil separates. Add lentils. Slowly bring lentil
mixture to the boil. Add freshly ground black pepper to
season. Add freshly chopped coriander. Add a swirl of
fresh cream. Serve with chapattis or naan bread.

CHANA MASALA

This dish is deliciously spicy and tangy. It's also packed full of protein, iron and folic acid.

Serves: 6
Cooking time: 40 minutes

Ingredients

1 tsp turmeric
2 tsp garam masala
2 tsp coriander seeds
1 tsp cumin seeds
2 cup chick peas, soaked overnight, boiled and drained
5 tbsp butter
3 cloves garlic
2 large onions, chopped
1 cup tomatoes, chopped
juice of 1 lemon
1/2 cup plain full-fat yogurt
2 tbsp coriander, chopped

Method

Blend dry spices to make a powder.
Blend garlic and ginger into a paste with a little water.

Set aside.

Heat butter in a large frying pan. Add onions. Cook on low heat until translucent, stirring occasionally. Add garlic and ginger. Cook 1 minute. Turn up heat. Add tomatoes. Saute on medium heat until tomatoes are soft. Add drained chick peas. Add 1/2 cup water. Bring to boil. Reduce heat to low. Simmer partially covered to allow water to evaporate. Simmer 20 minutes. Stir occasionally. Remove from heat. Add juice of 1 lemon. Cook for 1 minute. Remove from heat.

Stir in yogurt. Add chopped coriander. Cook 2 minutes more. Serve hot with pappadums.

RAJMAH

In this popular weekend brunch dish,
red kidney beans are cooked with onions
and tomatoes.

Serves: 6

Cooking time: 45 minutes

Ingredients

1 1/2 cups red kidney beans, soaked overnight

2 large onions, chopped

4 cloves garlic, peeled and chopped

5 large tomatoes, chopped

1 tsp cumin seeds

1 tsp turmeric

3 tbsp butter

8 cups cold water

1 tsp garam masala

black pepper, ground

Method

Drain the kidney beans. Place beans, onions and garlic in a large saucepan. Add water, tomatoes, cumin seeds, turmeric and butter. Cover pan. Cook 1 hour, or until beans are cooked. Add garam masala. Add a little black pepper to taste.

Simmer 5-10 minutes, uncovered until sauce thickens. Serve hot. Garnish with coriander leaves. Serve with jeera rice, plain rice or chapattis.

MCLEOD GANJ CHICKEN MOMOS

Minced chicken and Nepali spices are stuffed into a dough wrap.

Dough Wrappers

Ingredients

5 cups all-purpose flour

1 tbsp sunflower oil

1 cup cold water or as required

Filling

1 kg chicken, minced

1 cup onion, finely chopped

1/2 cup spring onion, finely chopped

1 tbsp garlic, minced

1 tbsp fresh ginger, minced

1/2 tsp Szechwan pepper

1/2 tsp nutmeg, grated

1/2 tsp turmeric

1 tbsp cumin powder

3 tbsp sunflower oil

ground black pepper

To make filling

Place all filling mixture into a bowl. Mix and adjust seasoning with freshly ground pepper. Cover and place in fridge for 1 hour.

To make dough

Place flour, oil and water into a bowl. Mix ingredients together. Place dough on floured board. Knead until a smooth texture. About 10 minutes. Cover with kitchen film and a clean towel. Leave for 15-30 minutes. Uncover and knead a second time until smooth and elastic. Break dough into 12 small pieces and roll each into a ball. Place one ball at a time onto a floured board. Roll out into a 10 cm circular shape. Repeat with remaining dough.

To fill dough

Place wrapper in left palm. Place 1 tbsp filling in the middle of the wrapper. With the right hand bring edges together to make a half circle with filling inside.

Pleat the edges. Then pinch and twist the pleats to make sure none of the filling escapes during cooking. Repeat until all 12 filling wrappers are ready to steam

To steam

Grease the steamer basket with oil to prevent dumplings from sticking. Place uncooked momos into the steamer. Place a lid on the steamer. Steam dumplings until they are thoroughly cooked, about 10-15 minutes. Remove from steamer and serve immediately. Serve on a plate with a dip (achar) of your choice. This recipe is for steamed dumplings, but you can also fry the dumplings.

SESAME TOMATO ACHAR FOR MOMOS

Achar is a Hindustani word for a spicy variety of pickle. Here is a classic Nepali recipe using sesame seeds.

Ingredients

2 large tomatoes

1 cup sesame seeds

1 cup coriander, chopped

1 tbsp garlic, minced

1 tbsp fresh ginger, minced

1 tsp cumin seeds

1 tbsp mustard seeds

2 tbsp lime juice

1 tbsp lime zest

black pepper to taste

Method

Place tomatoes on a baking tray. Drizzle with a little oil. Roast in hot oven 200 degrees C for 15-20 minutes until charred.

Remove skin and place tomato flesh in a bowl. In a frying pan heat sesame seeds, mustard and cumin seeds. Stir well until the seeds pop taking care not to burn. Remove from heat. Blend the seeds into a powder. Add tomatoes, chopped coriander, garlic, ginger, lime zest and blend to a smooth paste. Add a little cold water if too thick. Place achar in a serving bowl. Serve with steamed momos.

PORK-SHRIMP MOMOS
Shrimp, pork and spices, sealed in steamed or fried dumplings. A succulent, tasty snack.

Filling

500g shrimp or prawn, cleaned, de-veined, minced
500g pork, minced
1 cup onion, finely chopped
1/2 cup coriander, finely chopped
1 tbsp garlic, minced
1 tbsp ginger, minced
1/2 tsp Szechwan pepper
1/2 tsp nutmeg
1 tbsp curry powder
sunflower oil for cooking
black pepper, ground

To make filling

Place all filling mixture into a bowl. Mix and adjust seasoning with freshly ground pepper. Cover and place in fridge for 1 hour.

To make dough

Place flour, oil and water into a bowl. Mix ingredients together. Place dough on floured board. Knead until a smooth texture. About 10 minutes. Cover with kitchen film and a clean towel. Leave for 15-30 minutes. Uncover and knead a second time until smooth and elastic. Break dough into 12 small pieces and roll each into a ball. Place one ball at a time onto a floured ball. Roll out into a 10 cm circular shape. Repeat with remaining dough.

To fill dough

Place wrapper in left palm. Place 1 tbsp filling in the middle of the wrapper. With the right hand bring edges together to make a half circle with filling inside. Pleat the edges. Then pinch and twist the pleats to make sure none of the filling escapes during cooking. Repeat until all 12 filling wrappers are ready to steam.

To steam

Grease the steamer basket with oil to prevent dumplings from sticking. Place uncooked momos in the steamer. Place a lid on the steamer. Steam dumplings until they are thoroughly cooked, about 10-15 minutes. Remove from steamer and serve immediately. Serve on a plate with a dip (achar) of your choice. You can also fry these dumplings.

SWEET TAMARIND MANGO ACHAR FOR MOMOS

A sweet sour dip-sauce to serve with momos.

Ingredients

1 1/2 cup mangoes cut into small chunks

1 1/2 tbsp tamarind paste (no seeds)

1/2 cups brown sugar

1/2 tbsp garlic, minced

1/2 tbsp ginger, minced

1/2 tsp cumin seeds

1/2 tsp Szechwan pepper

black pepper to taste

Method

In a frying pan, heat cumin seeds. Stir well until the seeds pop taking care not to burn. Remove from heat. Add mangoes, garlic, ginger and tamarind paste and brown sugar. Mix well. Simmer on low heat for 30 minutes or until tomatoes are tender. Remove from heat. Cool. Puree tamarind mango mixture to a smooth paste. Add a little cold water if too thick. Place achar in a serving bowl. Serve with steamed momos.

TIBETAN STYLE MOMOS

A traditional recipe. These small, hand made dumplings are filled with pork and lamb.

Filling

500g minced lamb

500g minced pork

1 cup onion, finely chopped

1 cup cabbage, finely chopped

1 cup mushrooms, finely chopped

1 tbsp garlic, minced

1 tbsp ginger, minced

1/2 tsp Szechwan pepper

3 tbsp sunflower oil
black pepper, ground

To make filling

Place filling mixture into a bowl. Mix and adjust seasoning with freshly ground pepper. Cover and place in fridge for 1 hour.

To make dough

Place flour, oil and water into a bowl. Mix ingredients together. Place dough on a floured board. Knead until a smooth texture. About 10 minutes. Cover with kitchen film and a clean towel. Leave for 15-30 minutes. Uncover and knead a second time until smooth and elastic. Break dough into 12 small pieces and roll each into a ball. Place one ball at a time onto a floured ball. Roll out into a 10 cm circular shape. Repeat with remaining dough.

To fill dough

Place wrapper in left palm. Place 1 tbsp filling in the middle of the wrapper. With the right hand bring edges together to make a half circle with filling inside. Pleat the edges. Then pinch and twist the pleats to make sure none of the filling escapes during cooking. Repeat until all 12 filling wrappers are ready to steam.

To steam

Grease the steamer basket with oil to prevent dumplings from sticking. Place uncooked momos in the steamer. Place a lid on the steamer. Steam dumplings until they are thoroughly cooked, about 10-15 minutes. Remove from steamer and serve immediately. Serve on a plate with a dip (achar) of your choice. You can also fry these dumplings.

KASHMIR

Kashmir cuisine is elaborate and influenced by the Buddhist and Pandits (medicinal doctors who had the knowledge of herbs and spices). Kashmir cuisine is also influenced by Northern Indian, Persian and Central Asian cuisine. Mutton and chicken are the most notable ingredients. The dishes are often prepared with dried fruits, yogurt and spices.

DAHIWALA KORMA ANISE
A mild dish, chicken or lamb,
cooked in a creamy yogurt sauce.

Serves: 6

Cooking time: 1 hour 30 minutes

Ingredients

1 kg lamb or chicken, cubed

2 tsp aniseed powder

4 cardamom pods, crushed

1 tsp ginger powder

3 cloves

2 bay leaves

1 tsp black peppercorns

3 medium onions, finely chopped

1/2 tsp sugar

2 tsps garam masala

3 cups plain full-fat yogurt

sunflower oil

Method

Blend onions, ginger and garlic to a paste. Add 1 cup
yogurt. Marinate the meat in onion mixture for 1 hour.
Heat 3 tbsp of oil in a saucepan. Add lamb or chicken
and brown. Add 2 cups of water. Cover with lid. Lower

heat. Cook until meat is tender. Add aniseed, ginger, cloves and cardamoms. Add 2 cups yogurt. Cook until the meat absorbs the yogurt. Stir in garam masala. Serve hot with buttered wedges of naan bread.

HYDERABAD BIRYANI
A popular dish made with basmati rice, lamb or chicken.

Serves: 6
Cooking time: 1 hour

Ingredients for the meat

1 kg lamb, mutton or chicken breast, cubed

250g Greek style yogurt

2 large onions, cut thinly lengthwise

4-6 tsp ginger/ garlic paste

2 cloves

2 tsp coriander powder

1 tsp turmeric

1/4 tsp ground nutmeg

2 tsp garam masala powder

Ingredients for the rice

500g basmati rice

4 tbsp butter

2 bay leaves

1 tsp cumin seeds

2 cardamom pods

2 cm stick cinnamon

1/2 tsp saffron threads soaked in warm water (15 minutes)

1/2 cup chopped mint leaves (without stalks)

1/2 cup chopped coriander leaves

2 tbsp butter

Method

Cut meat into cubes. Add ginger/garlic paste and all the spices, herbs and yogurt for the meat marinade. Toss the meat until well coated. Cover and refrigerate overnight.

Wash rice and place in a bowl of water. Soak for one hour until the rice softens. Drain well.

In a large saucepan, heat butter. Add cumin seeds, cardamom pods and cinnamon sticks. Cook 15 seconds until aromatic. Add onions and fry until onions are fragrant and golden brown.

Stir in saffron, add water and simmer for 5 seconds. Add drained rice. Toss and coat with onions and saffron. Add 220mls water. Stir rice and then bring to boil. Cook 5 minutes. Remove from heat and set aside.

Heat oven to 180 degrees C. Butter a large pan. Add meat with marinade and spread over the bottom of the pan. Drizzle remaining 2 tbsp butter over meat. Add rice, spreading it over the meat. Cover pan with tin foil. Bake 1 hour until the rice is cooked and the meat is cooked and tender. Serve hot, topped with chopped mint leaves and accompanied by mango pickle and chutney.

MASALA SPICED CHICKEN CURRY

The spicey fragrant masala paste gets absorbed deep into the chicken.

Serves: 6 - 8
Cooking time: 1 hour

Ingredients:

1 1/2 kg chicken, skinned and cut into pieces
1 cup Greek style yogurt
1 tsp cumin seeds
3 tomatoes, roughly chopped

2 onions, sliced thinly and pre-fried till crisp
2 tbsp butter

Masala Paste

Ingredients

2 cm fresh ginger, peeled and sliced
6 cloves fresh garlic, peeled
1 tsp coriander powder
1/2 tsp fennel powder
1 tsp cumin seeds
3 cardamom pods
2 tbsp lime juice
pinch mustard powder

Method

Place all masala ingredients together in a food processor or blender and grind to a paste. Set aside.

Method

Put masala paste and yogurt in bowl. Mix thoroughly. Coat over the chicken pieces and keep aside in the fridge for 3 hours. Heat 2 tbsp butter and fry cumin seeds. Add tomatoes. Add chicken and paste. Add a little water. Cook over low flame until the chicken is cooked and there is no sauce. Serve chicken with fried onions to garnish or fried cashew nuts.

KASHMIRI PUMPKIN CURRY
A soft, sweet pumpkin curry, with cinnamon and cardamom flavors.

Serves: 6
Cooking time: 30 minutes

Ingredients

1 kg pumpkin, (or potato) peeled and cut into chunks

1 tsp garam masala

1 tsp cumin seeds

1 tsp turmeric

1/2 tsp garam masala powder

1 tbsp fennel/aniseed powder

1 1/2 tsp coriander powder

1/2 tsp ground cloves

2 cardamom pods

1 bay leaf

1 cinnamon stick

1 1/2 cup plain yogurt

2 tbsp cashew nuts, chopped
sunflower oil

Method

Prick the pumpkin (or potatoes) with a fork and soak for 20 minutes in water. Drain.

Heat oil over a medium flame. Fry pumpkin (or potatoes) until golden brown. Drain on paper towels and keep aside.

In another pan heat 2 tbsp oil and fry cumin seeds. Add the spices. Cook until golden brown. Add pumpkin and yogurt. Add 1/2 cup hot water. Cover and cook on low flame for about 10-15 minutes. Add a little more water if necessary. Serve hot with chapattis or naan.

KASHMIRI ROTI BREAD

Kashmiri roti, is a layered bread that reveals flavors of aniseed and butter.

Serves: 6 - 8
Cooking time: 30 minutes

Ingredients

500g finely ground wheat flour (aata)

3/4 cup warm water
1 tsp white sugar
1 1/2 tsp softened yeast
1 tsp aniseeds, crushed
pinch of salt (optional)
butter

Method

Dissolve sugar in warm milk and add softened yeast.
Mix with a fork. Sieve the flour onto a bench. Make a
well in the flour. Add aniseeds, salt, milk and 1 tbsp
butter and add yeast mixture.
Knead dough until soft and elastic. Cover with a damp
cloth. Leave in a warm place until double in size.
Divide into balls the size of a lime and roll into a ball.
Place the ball of dough onto a floured bread board and
roll out in a circle. Pick up the roti and quickly "clap"
between both hands to remove any excess flour and
prevent burning. Cook on a griddle, then brown over
a gas flame or open fire turning with long metal tongs.
Serve with hot melted butter.

PUNJAB

The people of the Punjab love their food and enthusiastically celebrate eating together. Punjab cuisine has a large range of tasty spicy vegetarian and non-vegetarian dishes. Onions, ginger and garlic are used extensively to enhance flavor.

LAMB WITH CHANA DAL

A tasty succulent lamb curry which features chana dal, (chick peas).

Serves 6 - 8

Cooking time: 1 hour 30 minutes

Ingredients

1 kg lamb or mutton, cut in cubes

1 tbsp garam masala powder

1 1/2 cup chana dal, soak in water 2 hours

2 large brown onions, chopped finely

4 tomatoes, skinned and chopped

1 tbsp fresh ginger, peeled and chopped

1 tbsp fresh garlic, peeled and chopped

1 cup plain yogurt

1 tsp turmeric powder

1 tbsp cumin powder

1 tsp sugar

1/2 bunch fresh coriander, washed and roughly chopped

1/2 bunch chopped mint

sunflower oil

Method

Wash chana dal. Soak for 1 1/2 hours. Drain. Cook chana dal in a covered pan with water until soft but still separate. Drain and keep aside.

Heat 5 tbsp oil in a saucepan. Add lamb and fry until browned. Blend ginger and garlic together into a paste. Add to the meat. Add spices. Blend onions and tomato to a paste and add to the meat. Cook on low heat until rich and aromatic. Add sugar and yogurt. Add 2 cups of water. Cover and simmer a further 30 minutes or until the meat is tender. Add chana dal and mix together. Simmer 5-10 minutes. Add mint and coriander leaves. Serve with naan or plain boiled rice.

PUNJABI LAMB KORMA
A really tasty Indian recipe that is very mild.

Serves: 8
Cooking time: 1 hour 30 minutes

Ingredients

1 kg lamb, cut in pieces
3 brown onions, thinly sliced
1 head of garlic, peeled and chopped
2 cm fresh ginger, peeled and chopped
1 bunch coriander, washed and chopped
1 bunch mint (no stalks) chopped
100g of shredded coconut
1/2 mango sliced
2 tsp garam masala
1 tsp turmeric powder
sunflower oil

Method

Blend ginger, garlic, mint and coriander leaves
together into a paste in a food processor. Marinate
the lamb in the spice, ginger and garlic paste for 30
minutes.
Fry onions until golden brown. Add marinated lamb.

Fry until aromatic. Add two cups of water, shredded coconut and mango. Cover and simmer until the meat is tender. Serve hot with steamed rice.

MASALA KEBAB

Chicken or lamb marinated in a special blend of spices.

Serves: 6

Cooking time: 1 hour 30 minutes

Ingredients for kebab

1 kg chicken (or lamb) minced

1 onion, chopped

1 tsp cumin powder

1 tbsp corn flour

Ingredients for masala paste

3 onions, sliced

4 tomatoes, sliced

1 tbsp fresh ginger paste

1 tbsp fresh garlic paste

1/2 tsp turmeric powder

1 tsp cumin powder

1 tsp coriander powder

1 tbsp coriander leaves, chopped

1 tbsp mint, chopped

1/2 tsp black pepper

1 tsp garam masala

2 tbsp fresh cream

sunflower oil

Method

Combine chicken (or lamb) with corn flour. Shape into small ovals with wet hands.

Set aside. Heat oil in a large pan. Add sliced onions. Cook until transparent. Add garlic/ginger paste and fry until brown (about 2 minutes). Add tomatoes and masala spice mix except garam masala powder and crushed black pepper. Cook the masala paste for 5 minutes. Add kebabs, cover and simmer on low heat for 15 minutes. Remove pan from heat. Add garam masala powder, pepper and cream and stir through. Serve hot. Serve with roti bread and raita.

GREEN PEA KOFTA CURRY

Pea paste is shaped into small balls, fried, then added to a delicious potato curry.

Serves: 4

Cooking time: 30 minutes

Ingredients

1/2 kg green peas, shelled and pureed

1 tsp poppy seeds

2 tbsp chick pea or plain flour

2 small onions, finely chopped

2 cloves

1 tsp cumin seeds

1 tsp turmeric

1 tsp coriander powder

1 tsp garam masala

2 large potatoes, peeled and cubed

1/2 cup fresh coriander leaves, chopped

sunflower oil

Method

Mix flour into the pea paste and add poppy seeds. Make into small balls and deep fry in hot oil until golden. Heat oil in a frying pan. Add onions, and cook until brown. Add cloves, cumin seeds, coriander powder, turmeric and garam masala. Cook until aromatic. Add potato cubes. Cook potatoes until tender. Add 1 cup of water. Cook on low heat until the sauce is thick. Add the pre-cooked koftas and simmer for 3-5 minutes. Serve hot with freshly cooked rotis.

PUNJAB FISH CURRY
A spicy tasty fish curry
cooked in the traditional way.

Serves: 6
Cooking time: 1 hour

Ingredients

500g fillets of fresh fish
2 onions, finely sliced
1/2 cup chick pea flour
2 tbsp lime juice
1/2 tsp saffron threads (optional) dissolved in 1 tsp

warm water

1 cm fresh ginger, peeled and sliced

1 cup coriander leaves, washed and chopped

1/4 tsp ground nutmeg

butter

sunflower oil

Masala Paste

Ingredients

2 cm fresh ginger, peeled and sliced

1/4 tsp ground cloves

5 green cardamom pods

4 tbsp coriander seeds toasted in a fry pan

1 tsp peppercorns

Method

Wash and dry fish fillets. Rub with flour. Process half the ginger and fresh coriander into a fine paste in a food processor. Rub this over the fish and leave to marinate. Wash the fish again. Marinate the fish in the remaining paste for 15 minutes. Wash fish and pat dry with kitchen paper.

Heat 4 tbsp butter in a pan. Fry onions until golden and crisp. Remove from pan and drain on kitchen paper. Fry fish in the onion butter with the masala paste. Add 2 tbsp lime juice and 3 tbsp water. Cover saucepan with lid. When the water has evaporated and the masala has separated from the butter, add the cooked onions, saffron and nutmeg. Cook a further minute.

Serve with fresh coriander leaves.

DELHI

The food of Delhi is legendary. It's a veritable taste explosion in the culinary hub of India. Especially the street food where many of the restaurants date back to the 1870's and 1880's. You can find old shops still serving original recipes for paranthas fried in cast-iron pans. Most Delhi dishes are served with chutneys such as mint, banana, tamarind and vegetable pickles.

SAFFRON CHICKEN CURRY

Rita's recipe for a delicious colorful saffron curry.

Serves: 8

Cooking time: 45 minutes

Ingredients

1 kg chicken, cut into 8-10 pieces

500g onions, finely chopped

500g potatoes, sliced

500g tomatoes, skinned and chopped

500g fresh green peas, shelled (or frozen)

1 tsp ginger and 1 tsp garlic (blended into a paste)

juice of 1/2 lime

1/2 tsp saffron threads, toasted

1 cup coriander leaves, roughly chopped

butter

Masala Paste

Ingredients

4 cloves fresh garlic

1 stick cinnamon (or 1 tsp cinnamon powder)

4 cloves

1 tbsp fresh ginger, finely chopped

1 tsp cumin seeds

Method for masala paste

Blend together in a food processor to a make an aromatic paste.

Method

Place chicken in a dish and mix the tomatoes and masala paste with the chicken.

Cover the chicken with garlic/ginger paste and onion. Bake in a 200 degree C oven. When half cooked, add lime juice. Cover the chicken with 2 tbsp butter. Add potatoes and vegetables mixed with saffron. Lower the oven temperature to 180 degrees C and roast until the vegetables are cooked. Garnish with coriander and serve with rice.

GURKHA
BEEF CURRY

An easy to make tender beef curry with a mixture of fragrant herbs and spices.

Serves 6

Cooking time: 30 minutes

Ingredients

500g beef, cut into cubes

2 large tomatoes

3 cloves

3 cardamom pods, crushed

3 curry leaves

1 cinnamon stick

2 bay leaves

1 tsp ginger paste

1 tsp garlic paste

2 large onions, finely chopped

1 tbsp mint leaves, washed and chopped

sunflower oil

black pepper to taste

Method

Heat oil in a large pan. Add onions and fry until

transparent. Add cardamoms, cinnamon, bay leaves, ginger, garlic, cloves and cook until aromatic. Add meat. Fry meat on low heat with onions and spices until brown. Add tomatoes, mint and mix. Add 1/2 - 1 cup water. Simmer covered until meat is cooked and makes a rich sauce. Serve hot with rice.

OLD DELHI RAILWAY STATION CURRY

A colonial lamb curry using fresh spices and herbs.

Serves: 6
Cooking time: 40 minutes

Ingredients

500g lamb or mutton, cut in cubes
6 black peppercorns
2 large brown onions, sliced
1 2cm cinnamon stick
3 cloves
4 green cardamoms, crushed
10 curry leaves

2 tsp fresh ginger, minced

2 cloves fresh garlic, finely chopped

2 tbsp sunflower oil

2 tbsp malt vinegar or tamarind paste

Method

Place lamb in a large bowl. Add ginger and garlic. Heat oil in a pan. Fry onions until golden brown. Add curry leaves, cinnamon, cloves, cardamoms and fry until brown. Add meat. Fry for 3 minutes. Add 1 cup water. Add vinegar (or tamarind paste) and simmer covered on medium heat until meat is cooked and the gravy is rich and brown. Serve with boiled rice and chutney.

RED FORT
CHICKEN CURRY

This chicken curry typically starts with spices cooked in hot oil. Very easy and delicious.

Serves: 6 - 8

Cooking time: 30 minutes

Ingredients

1 chicken, cut into serving pieces

2 large tomatoes, pureed

3 medium onions, chopped finely

1 tbsp garlic, finely chopped

1 tbsp ginger, minced

2 bay leaves

3 cloves

4 green cardamom pods, crushed

2 cm stick cinnamon

2 tbsp sunflower oil

1 tsp turmeric

500 ml hot water

Method

Heat oil in a pan. Add cinnamon stick, bay leaves, cloves and cardamom. Add onion and cook until golden brown. Add ginger and garlic and cook for 3 minutes. Add chicken pieces and cook for 5 minutes. Add turmeric powder and cook for a further 5 minutes while stirring. Pour 1 liter of hot water over the chicken and onion mixture. Bring to boil. Cover. Reduce heat and cook for 20 - 30 minutes. Remove lid. Add tomatoes. Simmer 5 minutes. Add a little water if necessary. Add a grind of black pepper to taste. Place in a serving dish. Serve hot with boiled rice, buttered naan bread and chutneys.

CONNAUGHT PLACE CURRY

A classic curry made with chunks
of lamb or mutton and potatoes.
A favorite from colonial times.

Serves: 6

Cooking time: 1 hour

Ingredients

500g lamb or mutton, cubed

500g potatoes, peeled

1/4 cup plain yogurt

2 bay leaves

1 cm cinnamon stick

1 cup coriander leaves, washed and chopped

1 tsp garam masala

Masala Paste

Ingredients

2 cloves garlic, peeled

1 tsp cumin seeds

1 tsp coriander powder

2 onions, chopped

3 large tomatoes, skinned and chopped

Blend all ingredients in a food processor, to make a paste.

Method

Heat butter in a saucepan and add potatoes cut into slices. Fry potatoes until golden. Put aside.

Fry the meat in the same pan and set aside. Next fry the masala paste mixture until aromatic and brown taking care not to burn. Add the meat and simmer in the sauce. Add yogurt and 1/4 cup of water. Add the potatoes, bay leaves and cinnamon stick. Add garam masala as the sauce thickens. Simmer on low heat. Add water as needed until the meat and potatoes are tender and cooked.

Add coriander leaves as a garnish.

SPICY EGG CURRY

A delicious potato curry made from boiled eggs cooked in a spicy tomato-onion sauce.

Serves 6

Cooking time: 40 minutes

Ingredients

6 medium potatoes

6 eggs, hard-boiled, shells removed

2 large onions

3 medium tomatoes

2 cloves garlic, finely chopped

1 tsp turmeric powder

1 tsp garam masala

1 tsp cumin powder

2 tbsp sunflower oil

4 curry leaves

Method

Heat oil in a large frying pan. Add onions and cook until transparent. Add curry leaves and garlic. Cook until brown and aromatic. Add tomatoes and fry for 5 minutes. Add turmeric, garam masala, cumin. Add 1/2 cup water. Bring to boil. Cook on low heat for 5 minutes. Cut eggs in half. Add to pan yolk side up.

Take care not to overturn or break the eggs. Simmer for 2-5 minutes until eggs are heated. Serve hot with rice.

LAMB CURRY WITH SPINACH
A rich lamb curry that features a creamy spinach sauce.

Serves 6 - 8
Cooking time: 1 hour

Ingredients

500g lamb or mutton
500g fresh spinach, finely chopped
(or use frozen spinach, cooked and drained)
butter
3 cardamom pods
2 cloves
4 black peppercorns, cracked
1 bay leaf
1/2 cup Greek style yogurt
pinch of bicarbonate of soda

Masala Paste

Ingredients

1 tsp cumin seeds

1 tsp coriander seeds

1 cm fresh ginger, peeled and chopped

2 onions, chopped

4 cloves fresh garlic, peeled

Blend all ingredients together in food processor to make a paste.

Method

Cook spinach in a small quantity of water with a pinch of bicarbonate of soda to preserve fresh green color. Blend in food processor. Set aside. Heat butter in a frying pan and add masala paste. Add meat, cardamoms, pepper, bay leaves and cloves. Cook meat until brown. Add spinach. Cook meat until tender. Reduce heat and add yogurt. Simmer for 5 minutes. Serve hot.

SHAHI KORMA

The aromatic paste of poppy seeds
and ginger brings added flavor to this dish.

Serves 6 - 8

Cooking time: 1 hour

Ingredients

1 kg lamb, cubed

1 cup plain yogurt

butter

12 almonds

4 peppercorns

2 cloves

4 cardamoms, crushed

1 tsp gara masala powder

1 stick cinnamon

1 bay leaf

Masala Paste

Ingredients

3 onions, chopped

3 cm fresh ginger, finely chopped

5 cloves garlic, peeled, finely chopped

2 tbsp poppy seeds (make sure they are fresh)
1 tsp coriander powder

Method

Heat 3 tbsp butter, add masala paste and fry together.
Add the ground masala powder.
Cook until butter separates from the spices, taking
care not to burn. Add the yogurt and cook on low heat.
Add meat and 1/2 cup of cold water. When meat is
browned, add 2 cups of cold water. Cover pan with
lid. Simmer until meat is tender in its own rich sauce.
Serve with rice.

CHICKEN BIRYANI

Tender chicken pieces in a creamy, spicy blend of onion, garlic and spices.

Serves: 8

Cooking time: 1 hour 20 minutes

Ingredients

1 chicken, cut into 10 pieces

300g basmati rice, washed

1 tsp coriander seeds

6 garlic, peeled and finely chopped

2 cm fresh ginger, peeled and minced

2 small onions, chopped

3 tbsp butter

2 cups yogurt

5 green cardamom pods

1 tbsp almonds, sliced

1 tbsp pistachios, shelled and sliced

1 tbsp fresh grated coconut (dried shredded or chopped)

1 tsp cumin powder

1 cup coriander, washed and chopped

1/2 tsp saffron (optional)

Method

Place chicken pieces in a large saucepan. Add water to cover. Add coriander seeds, garlic, and 2 tsp of chopped onion with the chicken. Bring to boil and simmer on low heat. Cook for 30 minutes until tender. Remove. Strain the stock and set aside.

Heat butter and fry onion until golden brown. Add chicken, yogurt, cardamom, cloves, almonds, pistachios, cumin seed powder and coconut. Add washed rice. Add chicken stock so it covers the ingredients. Add water if necessary so the liquid is 2 cm above the ingredients. Add saffron. Cover with a tight lid and simmer at a low temperature until the rice is cooked. Serve on a large platter with coriander leaves as a garnish and fried onions or shallots.

MATHURA POTATO CURRY

A quick, easy to make, simple curry.

Serves: 6

Cooking time: 45 minutes

Ingredients

6 medium potatoes, peeled and boiled

1/2 tsp ginger powder

1 tsp turmeric powder

1 tsp cumin seeds

1 cup coriander leaves, washed and chopped

Method

Mash potatoes. Heat 3 tbsp sunflower oil. Add cumin seeds. Add potatoes, ginger, turmeric. Add 1/4 cup water to make sauce. Take off heat and add coriander leaves.

PURIS

Hot puffed puris is a traditional
deep fried Indian bread

Ingredients

1 kg wheat flour
1/4 cup oil
oil for frying

Method

Sieve flour and add oil and enough water to make stiff
dough. Knead until soft. Make into balls the size of an
egg. Roll out into rounds on a lightly floured board.
Heat oil in pan. Pick up the dough between two hands
and quickly "clap" the circle to remove excess flour.
This prevents burning. Fry until golden brown.

BENGAL

Fish is the most dominant form of meat in the recipes of Bengal. There are more than 40 types of fresh water fish used in their recipes. Simple pulses are cleverly intensified by spices (such as mustard seed, fenugreek, aniseed and cumin). Bengali cuisine is about creating a balance of taste between the main ingredients and the seasoning.

BENGALI GOSH

A flavorful spicy meat curry
with fried turmeric potatoes.

Serves: 6

Cooking time: 1 hour

Ingredients

1.25 kg meat, cubed

3/4 cup plain yogurt

4 onions, sliced

2 bay leaves

2 tbsp ginger paste

3 tbsp garlic paste

2 tomatoes, cut in slices

3 large potatoes, peeled, cut in 4 pieces

6 tbsp oil

2 tsp fresh lemon juice

1 cup fresh coriander, chopped

1 tbsp turmeric powder

1 1/2 tsp dry roasted cumin seeds (blended to powder)

1/2 tsp mace powder

1/2 tsp nutmeg powder

1 cinnamon stick (2 cm)

5 cloves

5 green cardamom pods

1/2 tsp black pepper, coarsely ground

Method

Marinate potatoes in 1/2 tsp turmeric powder and set aside for 15 minutes.

Heat oil in a saucepan. Fry potatoes until they are golden brown. Drain and set aside. Fry onions in the same pan until they are golden brown. Add bay leaves, garlic and ginger pastes. Cook for 1 minute. Add turmeric, mace, nutmeg and coriander powder. Fry on medium heat for about 2 minutes. Add meat. Mix well and fry for 5 minutes. Add yogurt and tomatoes. Fold them in and fry until the oil leaves the spices. Add 2 1/2 cups warm water, cloves, green cardamoms and cinnamon to the meat mixture. Cover. Cook meat until brown. Cool. Add fried potatoes, roasted cumin seed powder, black pepper and lemon juice. Mix well. Bring to boil and cook on medium heat for 5-10 minutes. Garnish with coriander leaves.

BENGALI FISH CURRY
Spicy fish dish.

Serves: 6 - 8
Cooking time: 45 minutes

Ingredients

1 large fish cut into chunks
2 onions, peeled and sliced
2 large tomatoes, skinned and chopped
1 cup pumpkin, chopped in pieces
2 medium potatoes, chopped
1 tsp cumin seeds
1/2 tsp mustard seeds
1/2 tsp aniseeds
sunflower oil

Masala Paste

Ingredients

1 tsp mustard seeds
1 cm fresh ginger, sliced
1/2 tsp turmeric
Blend all ingredients together to make a paste.

Method

Heat 2 tbsp oil in a frying pan. Add fish and brown. Keep aside. Add the vegetables and masala paste. Add 1/4 to 1/2 cup water. When the vegetables are tender, remove with a slotted spoon. Heat 1 tbsp oil and fry cumin seeds and aniseeds for 1 minute. Add the vegetables back into the pan. Add the fish. Mix and cook for 3 minutes. Serve hot.

FISH KOFTA
Fried fish balls in a delicious, thick sauce.

Serves: 6
Cooking time: 1 hour

Ingredients

750g fish fillets
4 eggs
1 onion, finely chopped
1/2 tsp garlic and 1/2 tsp ginger (blended into a paste)
2 tsp turmeric
1 cup coriander leaves, washed and chopped
2 tsp finely chopped mint leaves
1/2 tsp cumin powder

1/4 tsp garam masala
sunflower oil

Masala Paste

Ingredients

2 onions
3 large tomatoes, skinned and chopped
1 tsp cumin
1 tsp garam masala
1/2 tsp turmeric
1 tsp white wine vinegar
a pinch of sugar

Method

Cook fish in milk. Mash with a fork. Add eggs, ginger
and garlic paste, turmeric and chopped onion. Using
wet hands, shape into balls the size of a lime. Fry in
hot oil until golden brown. Drain on kitchen paper.
Heat 2 tbsp of oil in a pan. Add masala paste. Fry
paste gently. Add fish balls and cook on low heat for
5 minutes. Serve hot with rice. Garnish with coriander
leaves.

BENGALI PRAWN CURRY

Marinated seafood with turmeric is characteristic of Bengali cooking.

Serves: 6

Cooking time: 30 minutes

Ingredients

500g prawns, shelled

1 tsp lime juice

1/2 tsp turmeric

1/2 cup pouring cream

1 cup fresh coconut milk

sunflower oil

Masala Paste 1

Ingredients

1 cm cinnamon stick

2 green cardamoms

1 bay leaf

2 black peppercorns

Blend to a paste.

Masala Paste 2

Ingredients

2 tsp cumin seeds
1 onion, chopped
1 cm ginger, peeled and finely chopped
1 pinch of sugar
Blend to a paste

Method

Squeeze lime juice over prawns. Leave 10 minutes.
Drain and pat dry with kitchen paper. Heat oil in a pan.
Fry prawns until pink. Add turmeric and masala paste
2 and fry for 5 minutes. Add masala paste 1. Mix and
add cream and coconut milk. Cook very slowly on low
heat for 8 minutes. Serve with rice.

MAHARASHTRA

The people in Maharashtra consider food equal to the creator of the universe and give thanks before eating. Fish, chicken, cashew nuts and coconut are widely used in dishes. The meals are eaten with traditional rotis made from rice flour, fermented rice or semolina.

KOLHAPUR CURRY

Kolhapur is a sleepy small town
famous for its mutton curry.

Serves: 6

Cooking time: 1 hour

Ingredients

500g - 750g meat, cubed (chicken, mutton or lamb)

1 tsp turmeric

2 tsp crushed garlic

1 tsp fresh ginger, grated

4 cloves

4 black peppercorns

1 tsp poppy seeds

1 tsp coriander seeds

1 tsp aniseeds

1 large onion, chopped finely

1/2 cup fresh coconut, grated

2 large tomatoes, skinned and chopped

6 medium potatoes, peeled and cut in halves

1 cup coriander leaves, washed and chopped (for
garnish)

Method

Place meat in a bowl and add ginger, garlic and turmeric. Leave to marinade in fridge for 2 hours. Heat 1 tbsp oil in a fry pan. Add poppy seeds, cloves, pepper, coriander seeds, and aniseeds. Cook together until aromatic. Add grated coconut and chopped tomatoes. Cook together until brown and aromatic. Take off heat and cool.

Heat 2 tbsp of oil in a heavy based saucepan. Add the marinated meat and sliced potatoes. Cook until golden brown. Add coconut mixture. Add 1/2 cup of water. Place lid on saucepan and simmer until meat is tender. Garnish with coriander leaves. Serve with rice or chapattis.

CURRY
WITH COCONUT SAUCE

This combination of coconut, onions and
tomatoes makes a unique curry.

Serves: 6

Cooking time: 30 minutes

Ingredients

500g meat

1/2 tsp turmeric

1/2 tsp garam masala

1 cup Greek style yogurt

1/2 cup cashew nuts

1 tbsp fresh ginger, blended into a paste

1 tbsp garlic, blended into a paste

1 tbsp fresh mint leaves, very finely chopped

4 black peppercorns

3 tsp coriander seeds

1 medium onion, chopped

1/2 fresh coconut, grated

3 large tomatoes, skinned and chopped

1 cup coriander leaves

Method

Place meat in a bowl. Add turmeric, garam masala, yogurt, cashew nut paste, ginger, garlic and mint leaves. Marinate for 1 hour.

Heat 1 tbsp oil in a fry pan. Add peppercorns and coriander seeds. Fry 1 minute. Add onions. Brown. Add coconut and brown. Take off heat and cool. Blend to a paste. Add tomatoes and coriander leaves. Blend together to make a paste.

In a heavy based saucepan, heat 2 tbsp oil. Add meat and marinade. Cook until brown. Add coconut paste and a little water. Bring to boil and cook for 30 minutes until the meat is tender. Serve hot with rice.

MAHARASHTRA CHICKEN CURRY

Tender chicken pieces in a red curry sauce.

Serves: 6 - 8

Cooking time: 1 hour

Ingredient

1 1/2 kg whole chicken, skinned and cut into pieces

2 onions, chopped

500g tomatoes, skinned and chopped

1/2 tbsp garlic, crushed

1/2 tbsp ginger, blended into a paste

2 cloves

1 cm cinnamon stick

2 tbsp malt vinegar

sunflower oil

Method

Place 1 chopped onion and 250g chopped tomatoes into a small saucepan. Add 1 cup water. Boil 10 minutes. Sieve together to create a red paste. Blend cloves, ginger, garlic and cinnamon together. Heat 2 tbsp oil in a saucepan and fry the remaining onions until golden. Take care not to burn. Add the cinnamon, blended paste, chicken pieces, remaining tomatoes and vinegar. Cook for 20 minutes and then add the red tomato and onion paste. Cook until the chicken is tender. Serve hot with rice.

CARAMEL CHICKEN CURRY
A subtle yet flavored curry.
Slowly caramelizing the chicken gives a deep, sweet flavour that infuses the curry.

Serves: 6

Cooking time: 40 minutes

Ingredient

1 1/2 kg chicken, skinned and cut into pieces

1 cup Greek style yogurt

1 tsp turmeric

1 tsp garam masala

4 cloves

4 peppercorns

1 tsp poppy seeds

1 tsp coriander seeds

1 tsp cumin seeds

3 large tomatoes, skinned and chopped

2 large onions, chopped

3 tbsp mint leaves

1/2 tbsp finely chopped garlic

1/2 tbsp fresh ginger, finely chopped

2 tsp sugar

2 tbsp coriander leaves, finely chopped

Method

Place chicken pieces in a bowl and add yogurt, garam masala and turmeric. Mix well. Marinate covered in the fridge for 2 hours.

Heat 1 tbsp oil in a fry pan. Fry peppercorns, poppy seeds, cumin seeds, coriander seeds until aromatic taking care not to burn. Add onions and cook until golden brown. Cool. Place in a food processor with tomatoes, ginger, garlic and mint leaves. Blend until a paste. Set aside.

Heat sugar in a saucepan with 1 tsp oil and cook until it caramelizes. Add 2 tbsp more oil and add the chicken pieces. Cook until brown taking care not to burn. Add tomato and spice paste that was set aside. Add a little water, if needed. Cover and cook on low heat, simmering for 20 - 30 minutes or until the chicken pieces are tender. Garnish with coriander leaves and serve with rice.

POTATO PURIS

Puris are an easy to prepare puffed spiced bread. Perfect as a snack, lunch or side dish.

Serves: 6

Cooking time: 45 minutes

Ingredient

250g potatoes, peeled and boiled

250g plain flour (sieved)

1 tsp garam masala

1 tsp cumin seeds

3 medium onions, minced

1 cup coriander leaves, washed and chopped

1 tbsp butter

sunflower oil

Method

Drain cooked potatoes. Place in a bowl. Mash potatoes. Add flour, cumin seeds, onions, butter, garam masala and coriander leaves. Mix together and knead into soft dough. Break off small balls and place onto a board dusted with flour. Roll out into small puris. Fry in hot oil until lightly brown. Drain on kitchen paper. Serve hot with sweet mango chutney.

GOA

Goan food has been influenced by many cultures due to it's proximity to the Christian world, the Arabic world and the Portuguese who settled there. However the main local Goan food is reflected in its tropical beach location and local village life where fish, chicken, pork and coconut are main features in Goan cuisine.

GOAN CHICKEN CURRY

This mild coconut and mango based curry
is spicy, rather than hot.

Ingredients

6 skinless chicken breasts, cut into 1 inch pieces

2 large onions, finely sliced

6 cloves garlic, blended into a paste

1 cm piece fresh ginger, blended into a paste

1 tbsp tamarind paste

1 bunch fresh coriander leaves

1 tsp poppy seeds

1 fresh coconut, grated

1 cup fresh mango, finely sliced

1 tsp lime juice

sunflower oil

Masala Paste

Ingredients

1 tbsp coriander seeds

1 tsp cumin seeds

6 black peppercorns

4 cardamom pods

1 cm cinnamon stick

1/4 tsp nutmeg, grated

1 tsp aniseeds

1 tsp cloves

1 tsp fenugreek seeds

Method

Heat 1 tbsp sunflower oil in a fry pan. Add spice blend ingredients and cook over medium heat. When aromatic, place in a blender or food processor and blend to a dry powder. Set aside.

Method

Add 1 tsp of oil to the fry pan and add onions. Cook until golden brown. Add half the grated coconut and all the poppy seeds. Fry until golden. Then process to a paste. Set aside.

Blend the milk from the other half of the coconut to get one cup of coconut milk. Add a little water if necessary. Set aside.

Heat 2 tbsp of oil in a large saucepan. Cook the other onion until brown. Add the chicken pieces with the masala paste and brown. Add mango and coconut milk. Stir. Place a lid on the pan and simmer until the chicken is cooked. Add lime juice and tamarind paste. Simmer 8 - 10 minutes. Serve with boiled rice.

GOAN PORK VINDALOO

A traditional tangy, spicy Goan pork dish.

Serves: 6

Cooking time: 45 minutes

Ingredients

1 kg pork, cubed

3 large potatoes

2 cloves

2 black peppercorns

2 cardamom pods

1 tsp sugar

1 large onion

2 tbsp malt vinegar

sunflower oil

Masala Paste

Ingredients

1 piece cinnamon

1 tsp cumin seeds

1 tsp coriander seeds

1 tsp turmeric powder

2 cloves garlic

1 cm piece fresh ginger

Blend to a paste in the food processor. Keep aside.

Method

Heat 2 tbsp oil in a fry pan and cook the potatoes until brown. Keep aside.

Fry the onions. Add pork with peppercorns, cardamoms, sugar and cloves.

Cook until brown. Add potatoes and masala paste and cook meat until it is tender. Add the vinegar and a little water. Simmer for 8 - 10 minutes. Serve hot with rice.

MANGO PRAWN CURRY

Prawns braised in a fragrant spiced mango, coconut sauce.

Serves: 6

Cooking time: 45 minutes

Ingredients

500g prawns, shelled

2 tbsp coconut or sunflower oil

1/2 small coconut

2 large onion, finely chopped

1 large ripe mango, peeled and sliced

Masala Paste

Ingredients

1 tbsp coriander seeds

1 tsp turmeric

1 tsp cumin seeds

1 green chilli, seeds removed (optional)

3 cloves fresh garlic, peeled

1 cm fresh ginger

Place in a food processor and blend to a paste.

Method

Prepare coconut as per the recipe in the front of this book. Wash prawns and dry on kitchen towels. Heat 2 tbsp oil in a fry pan. Fry onions until golden brown. Add the masala paste. Fry until brown. Add mango slices and 1 cup of water. Cook for 3 minutes. Add prawns with coconut milk and cook until prawns are tender. Take care not to overcook or prawns become tough. Serve hot with boiled rice.

GOAN MUSHROOM CURRY

Mushrooms cooked with Goan flavors.
Tangy, spicy and vibrant.

Serves: 4 - 6
Cooking time: 35 minutes

Ingredients

250g button mushrooms, wiped and cut quarters
1 small onion, finely chopped
1 large tomato, cut in quarters
1 cup fresh coconut, grated
2 cups water

1 tbsp sunflower oil
black pepper, freshly ground

Masala Paste

Ingredients

3 cloves garlic, peeled and finely chopped
2 cm fresh ginger, peeled and finely chopped
1 tsp tamarind paste (no seeds)
1 tsp cumin seeds
2 tsp coriander seeds
1 tsp turmeric powder

Method

Blend all masala paste ingredients together in a food
processor or blender until smooth, adding a little water
as necessary. Add grated coconut and blend again.
Set aside. Heat sunflower oil in a large saucepan.
Add onions and fry until golden brown. Add tomatoes
and cook for 3 minutes. Add mushrooms. Sauté until
water comes out of mushrooms and evaporates. Add
aromatic paste and fry for 5 minutes on medium heat.
Stir often. Add 2 cups of water (depending on the
consistency you prefer). Simmer 5 minutes. Serve hot
with rice.

GOAN DAL
WITH CHICKEN

A simple dal and chicken recipe high in flavor.

Serves: 6 - 8

Cooking time: 25 minutes

Ingredients for the dal

2 cups yellow moong/mung dal

6 cups water

1 tsp turmeric powder

1 large tomato

500g chicken breasts, cubed

Ingredients for the Coconut Paste

1 cup fresh coconut, grated or dry shredded coconut

1 medium onion, peeled and chopped

1 tbsp cumin seeds

5 cloves garlic, peeled and finely chopped

Method

Wash the dal beans. Cover and cook in a large saucepan with 6 cups water until tender.
Meanwhile blend coconut, cumin seeds and onions with a little water to make a smooth paste. Add

chicken, coconut paste to the dal. Add tomatoes. Simmer together to 20-25 minutes, until chicken is cooked, adding a little water if necessary and stirring occasionally. Note that this is a thicker style dal.

Ingredients for the tempering

1 tsp mustard seeds
1 tsp cumin seeds
2 curry leaves
2 cloves garlic, finely chopped
2 tbsp butter

Method

Heat butter in a fry pan. Add mustard seeds and cook until they "pop". Add cumin seeds to sizzle. Add crushed garlic and curry leaves. Fry until golden brown. Fry for 1 minute. Place dal in a serving bowl. Pour the tempering over the hot dal. Add a garnish of fresh coriander leaves. Serve with steamed rice.

GOAN
SPICED PORK SPARE RIBS
Slow cooked spiced pork ribs
from the shores of Goa.

Serves 4 - 6

Cooking time: 30 minutes

Ingredients

1 kg pork spare ribs

2 cloves garlic, finely chopped

1 tsp cumin powder

2 tsp coriander powder

2 tbsp sunflower oil

2 large onions, finely chopped

2 tsp sugar

2 tbsp vinegar

4 tbsp low-salt tomato sauce

Method

Place pork ribs in a bowl. Add coriander, vinegar, tomato sauce, cumin. Marinate 1 hour. Heat frying pan with oil. Cook onions and garlic until golden brown. Add marinated pork and stir well. Add 1/2 cup water. Cook on low heat until ribs are a rich brown color.

ANDHRA PRADESH

Andhra cuisine is influenced by the royal recipes of the Nawabs and its regional diversity. Traditional delicacies of this region have complex blends of spices. Recipes are mainly rice and chilli based, as Andhra Pradesh is the largest producer of rice and chillies in India. Many of the dishes are fiery. Pickles and chutneys are also very much an integral part of the meals.

NIZAMS KEBAB
Spicy meat roasted in the oven.

Serves 6 - 8
Cooking time: 1 hour

Ingredients

500g lamb, chicken breast or mutton, cut in cubes
2 small onions, sliced, fried crispy brown
1 cup fresh coriander leaves, chopped
1/2 cup Greek style yogurt
butter

Ingredients for tenderizing paste

1 tbsp garlic
1 tbsp ginger
1/2 cup fresh papaya or pineapple
Blend to a paste.

Masala Paste

Ingredients

12 almonds
1 tsp poppy seeds

1 tsp garam masala powder
Blend to a smooth paste

Method

Marinate meat in tenderizing paste for 2 hours.
Place on a baking tray. Mix yogurt with masala paste
spread over the meat cubes. Place onion and butter
over the kebabs and bake in a moderately hot oven
until well brown.
Serve hot with juices from roasting. Garnish with
coriander leaves if desired.

VEGETABLE KORMA

Royal vegetable korma. This is a richly spiced curry from the Nizam dynasty.

Serves: 8
Cooking time: 1 hour

Ingredients

200g French beans, chopped
200g cauliflower, broken into small florets
3 large tomatoes, chopped
4 potatoes, peeled and cubed
4 carrots, peeled and sliced
1 tbsp minced fresh ginger
1 tbsp minced fresh garlic
8 curry leaves
2 tsp garam masala
1 tsp turmeric
1 tsp cumin seeds
1/2 tsp mustard seeds
1 tsp raw sugar
1/2 cup seedless raisins
1 cup fresh coriander leaves, washed and chopped
sunflower oil

Method

In a large fry pan, heat 2 tbsp sunflower oil. Add mustard and cumin seeds and fry until they pop. Add onion garlic, ginger and curry leaves. Stir well until brown taking care not to burn. Add turmeric, vegetables, raisins, sugar and garam masala powder. If you don't have Kitchen King brand use another masala powder. Add 2 1/2 cups cold water and simmer on medium heat until vegetables are cooked. Place in a serving dish and garnish with coriander. Serve hot with rotis or naan bread.

GOLI KEBAB

Minced meat, spiced and fried.

Serves: 6 - 8
Cooking time: 1 hour

Ingredients

500g of minced meat (mutton, lamb, chicken or beef)
1 cup gram flour (chick pea flour) sieved (make sure it is fresh)
1 cup coriander leaves
1 cup mint leaves, washed (no stalks)
1 tsp garam masala
1 tsp turmeric
1/4 tsp bicarbonate of soda
sunflower oil

Method

Blend all ingredients in a food processor except oil and bicarbonate of soda.
Add bicarbonate of soda to the blended mixture.
Form into balls the size of large marbles. Heat oil in a pan. Fry goli in batches until golden brown. Drain on kitchen paper. Serve hot with chutney, fried onion rings and sliced fresh bread

CHICKEN MINT CURRY

Shredded chicken breast cooked in a rich onion and tomato sauce.

Serves: 6

Cooking time: 1 hour 30 minutes

Ingredients

1 kg chicken breast, skinned, cooked and meat shredded

1 tsp fresh ginger paste

1 tbsp mint leaves (no stalks), chopped

2 onions, finely chopped

3 medium tomatoes, finely chopped

1 tsp garam masala

1 cup coriander leaves (for garnish)

sunflower oil

Method

Heat 2 tbsp oil in a fry pan. Add ginger and onions and fry until golden brown taking care not to burn. Add tomatoes. Stir until the onions and tomatoes are cooked. Add shredded chicken. Cook until the oil separates from the meat.
Garnish with fresh coriander leaves. Serve with rotis or boiled rice.

DHAL OF RED LENTILS WITH ONION RAITA

Lentils served with a cooling onion, mint and coriander raita.

Serves: 4

Cooking time: 20 minutes

Ingredients

250g red lentils

1 tsp turmeric powder

sunflower oil

1 medium onion, peeled and grated

2 cloves garlic, peeled and finely chopped

1 tsp garam masala

Method

Wash lentils and place in a saucepan with turmeric. Cover with water 2 cm over the lentils. Simmer for 20 minutes until lentils are tender, adding more water if needed. Heat 2 tsp oil in a fry pan. Add onions and garlic. Cook for 1 minute. Stir in garam masala. Cook for 2 minutes. Add cooked lentils. Stir well.

Onion Raita

Ingredients

1 small red onion, finely sliced

1 handful mint leaves, stalks removed, chopped

1 handful coriander leaves, stalks removed, chopped

200 ml Greek style yogurt

Method

Place onions in a bowl. Add mint, coriander and yogurt. Mix well. Place in serving dish and chill before serving as side dish.

ROYAL RICE

A celebration dish with a royal combination
of rice, chicken, saffron, fruit and nuts.

Serves: 6 - 8

Cooking time: 40 minutes

Ingredients

2 cups long grain rice, rinsed well and drained

500g boneless chicken breast, skinned and cubed

2 cups Greek style yogurt

1/2 tbsp garlic, finely chopped

1/2 tbsp ginger, finely chopped

4 cloves

6 black peppercorns

8 green cardamom pods, crushed

1/4 cup pistachio nuts, chopped

1/4 cup slivered almonds, chopped

20 red or green grapes, seedless or seeds removed

20 pieces of pineapple, fresh or tinned, cut in small
chunks

1/2 tsp saffron soaked in 2 tsp milk

sunflower oil

4 tbsp butter

Method

Melt butter in a large saucepan. Fry onion in the butter until golden brown taking care not to burn. Add chicken and brown. Add cardamoms, peppercorns, cloves, yogurt, ginger and garlic, almonds, pistachios, raisins and saffron. Add water to cover. Cook covered with a lid on low heat, until the chicken is almost tender. Remove lid. Add washed and drained rice. Pour 4 cups of hot water over the rice and cover with a lid. Cook until the rice is done. Place rice and meat on a serving platter. Use grapes and pineapple as garnish. Serve hot.

KARNATAKA

This region has a diverse range of regional influences. In the north it's influenced by the Maharashtra. In the south Udupi cuisine. In the west, tasty seafood specialties and pork curries. In the hilly regions, tangy, spicy meat curries of pork, chicken and mutton.

MADRAS MEAT CURRY

Meat simmered in a rich curry sauce makes
this delicious curry world famous.

Serves 6 - 8

Cooking time: 1 hour

Ingredients

1 1/2 kg of meat, (lamb, beef or pork) cubed

4 onions, finely chopped

6 large potatoes, peeled and halved

1/2 tbsp ginger, finely chopped

1/2 tbsp garlic, peeled and finely chopped

1/2 tsp ground black pepper

1 tsp turmeric

1 tsp fennel seeds

1/4 tsp mustard seeds

1 tbsp coriander seeds

2 tbsp tamarind pulp

1 cm piece cinnamon

1 tbsp sesame seeds

4 cloves

1 tbsp poppy seeds

1 small coconut, grated

sunflower oil

Method

Place meat in a large bowl. Add the ginger, garlic, turmeric and pepper. Set aside to marinate for 2 hours. Make coconut milk using the recipe in the back of this book. Set aside.

Heat 1 tbsp oil in a fry pan and fry half the chopped onions. Add coconut, coriander seeds, cinnamon, poppy seeds, sesame seeds and cloves.

Brown together. Cool. Blend to a powder in a food processor. Set aside.

Heat 3 tbsp oil. Add remaining onions. Fry until golden. Add meat and potatoes. Add 3 - 4 cups of water. Cover and simmer on low heat until the meat and potatoes are cooked. Add the coconut paste, tamarind pulp and the coconut milk. Simmer for 10 - 20 minutes until the flavors are aromatic and blended together. Serve hot with boiled rice.

MEAT PULAO
A rice and meat dish
with a cashew nut base.

Serves: 6 - 8

Cooking time: 1 hour

Ingredients

2 cups rice, washed and drained

500g minced meat (lamb, beef or mutton)

1/2 cup grated coconut, blended

3 medium onions, peeled and chopped finely

6 black peppercorns

1/2 cup cashew nuts, roasted

sunflower oil

Masala Paste

Ingredients

1/2 tsp fenugreek seeds

1 tsp turmeric powder

1 tsp poppy seeds

1 tsp cumin seeds, toasted

1 tsp fresh ginger, finely chopped

1 tsp fresh garlic, finely chopped

1 small onion, peeled and finely chopped
Blend all together to make a smooth paste.

Method

Heat 3 tbsp oil in a large fry pan. Add black peppercorns. Add drained rice and stir for 3 minutes over low heat. Add 4 cups hot water. Bring to boil and turn heat down. Simmer on low heat until rice is almost cooked. Remove from heat. Heat 3 tbsp sunflower oil in a saucepan. Add onions and stir until transparent and golden. Add masala paste and mince meat. Cook on medium heat until the meat is cooked. Place meat mixture on a baking tray. Add rice and coconut paste to the mince. Bake in a hot oven 200 degrees C, until cooked. Serve hot with naan bread, pickles and chutney.

SPICY EGGPLANT CURRY

A delicious curry with the sweetness
of eggplant.

Serves 4 - 6

Cooking time: 25 minutes

Ingredients

4 eggplants, cut in quarters

2 onions

1/2 tsp cumin seeds

1/2 tsp garam masala

8 fresh or dried curry leaves (or 1 tsp curry powder)

1/2 tsp turmeric powder

1/2 coconut, grated

1 cup fresh coriander leaves, washed and chopped

1/2 lime or lemon juice

12 cashew nuts

sunflower oil

Method

Heat 2 tbsp oil in a large saucepan. Fry cumin seeds.
Add onions. Fry until golden. Add the eggplants,
garam masala, turmeric and cashews. Stir and cook
over medium heat for 5 minutes. Add a little hot
water and simmer for a further 10 minutes until the

eggplants are cooked. Squeeze lemon or lime juice to taste. Sprinkle with chopped coriander leaves. Serve hot with rice.

TAMIL NADU

Tamil Nadu has a belief that serving food is a service to humanity. The Tamil are famous for their hospitality. The flavors in this region are made from blending spices of ginger, coriander, garlic, cinnamon, nutmeg, coconut, mustard, pepper and coconut. Many traditional dishes are still made in a time honored way of elaborate preparation, then served on fresh green banana leaves, as it has been for centuries.

TAMIL
GREEN CHICKEN CURRY

Fresh coriander leaves add pungency to this simple chicken dish.

Serves: 6 - 8

Cooking time: 1 hour

Ingredients

1.5 kg chicken, cut into 6 - 8 pieces

2 onions, chopped

1 coconut, grated

1 tbsp tamarind pulp

1 tsp turmeric

2 tsp ginger, finely chopped

2 tsp garlic, finely chopped

2 cups fresh coriander leaves, washed and chopped

1 tbsp fine white flour

sunflower oil

Method

Heat 3 tbsp oil in a large saucepan. Add onions and cook until golden brown taking care not to burn.
Add chicken, garlic, ginger, tamarind, coriander and turmeric. Cook over medium heat for 7 minutes. Add 2

cups of cold water. Stir well. Cover and cook until the chicken is tender. Blend coconut and make coconut milk (follow the recipe for coconut milk, at the end of this book). Take coconut milk and whisk flour into it. Add this coconut mixture to the curry. Simmer for 10 minutes. Serve hot.

MIXED VEGETABLE CURRY

Bananas and cashew nut base gives this vegetable curry a sweet nutty flavour.

Serves: 6 - 8
Cooking time: 25 minutes

Ingredients

200g fresh or frozen peas
2 carrots, peeled and cubed
2 bananas, peeled and chopped
2 large potatoes, peeled and cubed
200g French beans (fresh or frozen)
200g of cabbage, shredded
8 curry leaves or 1 tsp curry powder
1 tsp turmeric
1 tsp cumin seeds

12 cashews

1 cup Greek style yogurt

Masala Paste

Ingredients

2 tsp cumin seeds

1/2 tsp black pepper

2 tsp rice

1 tsp poppy seeds

1/2 coconut, grated

Blend all the ingredients to make a paste.

Method

Cook the vegetables with cashew nuts in a little water.
Add turmeric. Drain in a sieve and keep the cooking
water aside.

Place yogurt in a bowl. Add masala paste. Mix well.
Add to the cooked vegetables together with the
vegetable cooking water.

Add 2 tbsp oil to a heavy based saucepan. Add curry
leaves and cumin seeds until aromatic. Pour over the
curry and mix through taking care not to break the
vegetables. Serve hot with naan bread.

SWEET SOUR CURRY
Slow cooking is the secret to this fragrant dish.

Serves: 6 - 8
Cooking time: 30 minutes

Ingredients

1 kg meat (pork, lamb, beef or mutton) cubed
2 tbsp vinegar
3 medium onions, chopped
1 cm ginger, finely sliced
6 cloves garlic, crushed
2 tbsp peanuts, crushed
1 tbsp coriander seeds
3 black peppercorns
'3 green cardamom pods, crushed
2 cm cinnamon stick
2 tbsp raisins
1 tsp cumin seeds
butter

Method

Fry meat until brown in 2 tbsp oil. Add 1/2 cup water.
Cover and cook on low heat for 25 minutes. Remove
from heat. Add vinegar. Set aside to marinate for 1

hour.

Blend all the spices, nuts and raisins together in a food processor.

Place 4 tbsp butter in a frying pan. Fry the onions until golden brown. Add the spices and fruit mixture. Cook for 3 minutes. Add the meat and brown. Simmer covered on low heat until the meat is cooked (length of cooking time depends on the meat). Serve hot with boiled rice and chutney.

NADU FISH CURRY

Fish and coconut go together perfectly
with ginger, garlic and spices.

Serves: 6
Cooking time: 45 minutes

Ingredients

500g fish fillets, sliced
1/2 small coconut, grated
1 tsp fresh ginger, finely chopped
4 cloves garlic, finely chopped
1 medium onion, finely chopped
6 curry leaves or 1 tsp curry powder

1 tsp turmeric

1 tsp coriander powder

1 tsp cumin powder

sunflower oil

Method

Make coconut milk. Add 1 tbsp oil to a saucepan. Fry onions, ginger, garlic, turmeric, coriander powder, cumin powder and curry leaves in hot oil until aromatic and brown. Add coconut milk and fish pieces. Turn down heat to low. Simmer until the fish is cooked. Take care not to boil. Serve with rice.

SIDE DISHES

Ideal for starters, snacks
or as a condiment for curries.

MANGO CHUTNEY

Serves: 6

Cooking time: 15 minutes

Ingredients

2 large ripe mangoes, peeled

1/2 tsp fennel seeds

1/2 tsp mustard seeds

1/2 tsp cumin seeds

1/2 tsp nigella seeds

2 tbsp sugar

1 tsp sunflower oil

2 cm fresh ginger, peeled and grated

1/4 tsp garam masala powder

1/2 bunch coriander leaves, washed

Method

Chop mangoes. Roughly chop coriander leaves
(no stalks). Heat oil in a saucepan. Fry spices until
aromatic. Add ginger and fry for 1 minute. Add
mangoes. Add garam masala. Stir well. Simmer for
3 minutes on low heat. Add sugar. Stir well. Add
chopped coriander leaves. Cook for a further 3
minutes taking care not to overcook or the mixture

will become too thick. Place chutney in serving bowl. Use with curries as a condiment or as a dip. Keep in a sealed container in the fridge for up to 4 days.

MINT CORIANDER RAITA

Serves: 4
Cooking time: 10 minutes

Ingredients

1/2 cup mint leaves
1/2 cup coriander leaves
1 onion finely chopped
1 tsp toasted cumin seeds
1/2 tsp chaat masala powder
1 cup plain yogurt

Method

Blend mint, coriander in a little water. Add onion, spices and yogurt. Stir. Place in serving bowl. Chill.

ONION TOMATO RAITA

Serves: 4

Cooking time: 10 minutes

Ingredients

1 cup plain yogurt

1 small red onion, chopped finely

1 large tomato, finely chopped

2 tsp mint leaves, washed and finely chopped

1/2 tsp cumin powder

coriander and mint leaves (for garnish)

Method

Place onion, tomato and mint in a bowl. Add yogurt.
Add dry spices. Mix. Garnish with fresh herbs.

BEETROOT AND CARROT RAITA

Serves: 4

Cooking time: 5 minutes

Ingredients

2 cups plain yogurt

1 medium beetroot, peeled, grated

1 medium carrot, peeled, grated

1 small onion, finely chopped

1 tsp cumin powder

Method

Place yogurt in a bowl. Add onions, carrot and beetroot. Add cumin. Mix well.

QUICK HUMMUS

Serves: 6

Cooking time: 5 minutes

Ingredients

2 cans low salt chick peas

1/4 cup olive oil (add more if needed)

4 garlic cloves, peeled

1/2 tsp black pepper, ground

1 tsp cumin powder

1/2 cup tahini paste

juice 1/2 lemon

1/2 small bunch fresh parsley, washed

Method

Place drained chick peas, spices, parsley and garlic in a food processor. Add tahini, lemon juice and olive oil. Blend until smooth. Serve with warm pita bread.

MINT CHUTNEY

Makes 1 bowl

Preparation time: 15 minutes

Ingredients

1/2 cup plain yogurt

1 cup mint leaves

1 cup coriander leaves

1 small red onion, peeled and chopped

1 cm fresh ginger, finely chopped

3 cloves garlic, peeled, finely chopped

1 tsp garam masala powder

1 tsp cumin powder

1 tsp mango powder (optional)

black pepper, ground

Method

Mix yogurt with spices. Blend mint and coriander leaves with fresh ginger and onion. Add a little water to make a smooth paste. Mix the green puree with the yogurt. Blend together. Serve with naan bread as a snack or with curries.

SWEET MANGO CHUTNEY

Serves: 4

Cooking time: 10 minutes

Ingredients

2 ripe mangoes, peeled and chopped

1 cup fresh coconut, or desiccated coconut

2 cloves garlic, crushed

1 cm tamarind

a little sugar

Method

Blend coconut with garlic and tamarind with a little water to make a paste. Place in a bowl. Add a little sugar to taste. Add chopped mangoes and mix together.

TOMATO PICKLE

Serves: 4 - 6

Cooking time: 30 minutes

Ingredients

4 large ripe tomatoes

1 tsp tamarind paste (no seeds)

2 cm fresh ginger, finely chopped

1/2 tsp mustard seeds

1 tsp cumin seeds

10 curry leaves

1 tsp turmeric powder

2 tbsp sunflower oil

Method

Place tomatoes and tamarind paste in a blender. Puree until smooth. Heat oil in a fry pan. Add cumin seeds. Fry until they "pop". Add chopped ginger. Fry until brown on a low heat. Add curry leaves. Fry for 2 seconds on low heat. Add tomatoes and tamarind paste. Stir well. Simmer on low heat for 5 minutes. Cool. Place in a clean, dry, airtight jar. Store in fridge for up to 5 days.

CORIANDER CHUTNEY

Makes: 1 bowl
Preparation time: 10 minutes

Ingredients

1 cup fresh coriander leaves, chopped
1 cm fresh ginger, finely chopped
1 - 2 tsp lemon juice
1 tsp cumin powder
black pepper, freshly ground

Method

Blend ingredients together with a little water to make a smooth paste. Add more lemon juice as necessary for taste. Store covered in the fridge. Use as an appetizer dip with breads or serve with curries.

SESAME COCONUT CHUTNEY

Makes 1 bowl
Preparation time: 15 minutes

Ingredients

1 cup coconut, freshly grated or desiccated
4 tbsp sesame seeds, roasted
3 tbsp peanuts, roasted
1 tbsp tamarind pulp (no seeds)
3 cloves garlic, peeled

Method

Roast peanuts in a pan. Roast sesame seeds in another pan.
Place all ingredients in a blender or food processor.
Add a little water and blend to a smooth paste.
Serve with breads or curries or on a dosa plate as an accompaniment.

JUST DESSERTS

MANGO MOUSSE

Serves: 6
Preparation time: 10 minutes

Ingredients

3 mangoes, chopped
1 cup thick cream
3 tbsp liqueur of your choice (optional)
1 tbsp sugar

Method

Place mangoes, liqueur and sugar in a blender. Blend until smooth. Whip cream and slowly fold in the mango mixture. Spoon into dessert bowls or tall glasses. Chill for 30 minutes.

BANANA AND GUAVA BREAD

Serves 6 - 8

Cooking time: 40 minutes

Ingredients

4 ripe medium sized bananas

2 ripe pink guavas, seeds removed, (optional)

1 1/2 cup all purpose flour

3 eggs

1/2 cup sugar

1/2 tsp baking soda

1 tsp baking powder

1 tsp pure vanilla extract

1/2 cup sunflower oil

Method

Heat oven to 180 degrees C. Grease and lightly dust a loaf pan with flour. Mash bananas with a fork. Cut guavas into quarters. Add to bananas. Sift flour, baking powder and baking soda. Place eggs, sugar and oil in a bowl. Whisk until creamy. Add bananas and guavas and mix again. Add flour to mixture. Pour into a loaf pan or cake tin. Bake 45 minutes until a skewer inserted in the middle comes out clean. Remove from tin. Cool on a rack. Serve warm or cold with butter.

JEWELED RICE PUDDING

Serves: 6
Cooking time: 20 minutes

Ingredients

2 cups leftover cooked basmati rice
4 cups milk
3 tbsp sugar
1/2 tsp cinnamon
1/2 tsp cardamom powder
2 tbsp almonds
2 tbsp raisins
2 tbsp unsalted pistachios

Method

In a large saucepan, mix rice, sugar, milk together. Cook on medium heat stirring all the time. Add cardamom and cinnamon after 5 minutes. Lower heat and cook for 15 minutes, stirring every few minutes until the rice thickens. When the rice is thicker, add almonds, pistachios and raisins. Remove from heat and add a little cream and/or a tsp of rosewater. Serve hot or cold in small bowls.

FRUIT PANCAKES

Serves: 6
Cooking time: 30 minutes

Ingredients

1 cup flour
1 cup milk
1 egg
1 egg yolk
1 tbsp melted butter
butter for cooking
Choice of bananas, mangoes, cooked apples, berries
sugar to taste

Method

Prepare fruit of your choice for the pancake filling as follows:

Banana Pancake

Slice bananas and add a little cinnamon and sugar.

Apple Pancake

Stew sliced apples with a little water, honey and cardamom pods.

Mango Pancake

Slice fresh mangoes and add a squeeze of fresh lime and a little sugar to taste.

Berry Pancake

Poach berries in a small pan until juice runs freely. Add a little sugar and cook to a syrup.

Lemon Sugar Pancake

Take one lemon and cut in wedges. Squeeze over cooked pancake and sprinkle with sugar.

Garnish

Whip some cream and sweeten with a few drops of pure vanilla and a little castor sugar. Use to garnish pancake.

Method

Place all ingredients except butter and fruit in a blender or food processor. Blend to a smooth batter. Set aside for 30 minutes. Melt 1 tbsp butter. Cool and add to the pancake mixture. Heat some butter in a non stick pan. Pour in a thin coating of pancake mixture. Tilt pan until the bottom is coated. Cook until the bottom of the pancake is golden. Turn over and cook the other side. Keep warm in the oven. When all pancakes are cooked, take filling and place in middle of each one. Roll each pancake up into a cylinder. Serve with a little cream.

FRUIT CUSTARD

Serves: 4
Cooking time: 30 minutes

Ingredients

2 1/2 cups milk
4 tbsp raw cane sugar
2 tbsp custard powder
4 tbsp milk taken from the 2 1/2 cups milk.
2 cups mixed seasonal fruit

Method.

Mix custard powder with 3 tbsp cold milk to make a smooth paste. Set aside. Warm the remaining milk taking care not to over heat. Add sugar to warmed milk and stir until dissolved. Add custard paste and cook on low heat until the mixture thickens. Stir continuously to avoid lumps and the mixture sticking to the bottom of the saucepan. Take off heat and cool. Peel and chop fruits of your choice. Add to cooled custard. Mix through and serve in bowls. Decorate with toasted shreds of coconut. Custard can be chilled in the fridge.

MANGO HALVA

Serves: 4 - 6
Cooking time: 30 minutes

Ingredients

1 cup semolina
1 large mango, chopped and blended
2 tbsp butter
1/4 - 1/2 cup sugar
250 ml milk
275 ml water

dried fruits : apricots, raisins, almonds

4 green cardamom pods, ground (husks removed)

a pinch saffron powder

Method

Heat butter in a heavy bottomed pan and add semolina cooking until it is golden. Add your choice of dried fruits and fry for 3 minutes. In another pan, heat 1 1/2 cups water. Add semolina and stir well. Add milk. Add sugar to taste. Stir on low heat until semolina absorbs the liquids. Add mango puree. Stir well until the liquid is reduced to make a paste. Add cardamom and saffron. Cover with a lid and cook for 2 minutes. Serve hot, warm or cold, garnished with pomegranate seeds (optional) or a swirl of thin pouring cream and toasted slivers of almonds.

TIBETAN RICE PUDDING WITH ROSE WATER

Serves: 6

Cooking time: 30 minutes

Ingredients

4 cups milk

1/2 cup rice

1/4 cup raisins

1/2 cup sugar

1 tsp cardamom seeds

1/4 cup blanched almond slivers

6 - 8 drops rosewater

1/2 cup water

Method

Wash rice and soak for 30 minutes in water. Place rice and water in a saucepan. Cover with lid. Cook until water evaporates. Add milk to rice and simmer on low heat, stirring occasionally for 30 minutes. Mash rice while cooking. When rice is creamy, add sugar and stir. Remove from heat and add crushed cardamom seeds, slivered almonds and rose water.

BANANA FRITTERS

Serves: 4 - 6
Cooking time: 30 minutes

Ingredients

200g plain flour
3 ripe bananas, mashed
1 tbsp sugar
1 cup milk
1/2 cup cold water
1/2 tsp pure vanilla essence
sunflower oil for frying

Method

Place dry ingredients in a bowl. Slowly add milk and water. Whisk to get a smooth batter. Add vanilla and mashed bananas. Beat well. Heat oil. Fry fritters until golden brown. Serve hot with ice cream.

CARDAMOM RICE PUDDING

Serves: 6
Cooking time: 1 hour

Ingredients

1 1/2 cups of long grain rice, washed
1/2 cup sugar
1 tsp cinnamon
1/2 cup almonds, sliced
1/2 cup pistachios, sliced
1/2 cup raisins
1 tsp cardamom powder
1/4 cup butter

Method

Wash rice. Soak in a bowl for 10 minutes and drain.
Dry on paper towels.
Melt butter in a large saucepan. Add rice, cinnamon
powder, raisins, nuts and cardamom. Fry on low heat
for 5 minutes. Add hot water to 2 cm above the rice.
Stir in sugar and mix well. Cover with a tight fitting lid
and cook on low heat, stirring occasionally until the
rice is cooked. Serve hot as a dessert with a swirl of

cream on the top and a sprinkle of toasted nuts. A little honey or rosewater can be added to this pudding just before serving.

MANGO COCONUT PUDDING

Serves: 6
Cooking time: 1 hour

Ingredients

6 ripe mangoes
1/2 coconut, grated
1/4 cup sugar
1 tsp cardamom powder

Method

Wash and peel mangoes and remove pip. Cut into medium pieces. Mix mango with sugar and cardamom powder. Blend coconut and strain the milk. Add to mangoes. Mix and place in a serving bowl. Chill in fridge. Serve in small bowls.

BEVERAGES

STREET LEMONADE

Serves: 2
Preparation time: 5 minutes

Ingredients

1 large lemon, cut in half
2 cups water
1/2 tsp cumin powder (optional)
sugar to taste
5 mint leaves, crushed
ice cubes

Method

Squeeze lemons and add to 2 cups cold water. Add sugar, cumin powder and stir until sugar dissolves. Pour into glasses and add ice cubes and mint.

MASALA (CHAI) TEA

Cooking time: 15 minutes

Ingredients

3 cups water
1/2 cup milk
2 black peppercorns
2 green cardamom pods
small 1 cm piece cinnamon stick
pinch green fennel seeds (optional)
2 cloves
1/4 tsp ground ginger
2 tbsp black tea leaves
sugar to taste

Method

Crush cardamom pods and cinnamon, or use coffee
grinder. Add spices to saucepan. Add water, ginger
and pepper and bring to boil. Remove pan from heat
and brew for 4 minutes. Add milk and sugar to pan.
Bring to boil. Remove from heat and add tea. Let brew
for 3 minutes. Stir. Strain chai into a warm teapot.
Pour into cups.

INDIAN GINGER TEA

Serves 4 - 6

Preparation time: 10 minutes

Ingredients

4 cups water

3 tea bags, black tea

1 cm fresh ginger, peeled and grated

4 green cardamom pods

3/4 cup milk

6 - 8 tsp raw sugar, to taste

Method

Place water, ginger, crushed cardamom pods in a saucepan. Bring to boil. Simmer for 5 minutes. Add sugar. Simmer 3 minutes. Add tea bags. Simmer 3 minutes. Add milk. Simmer for 2 minutes. Strain tea into cups. Serve hot.

MANGO BANANA SMOOTHIE

Serves: 4

Preparation time: 15 minutes

Ingredients

2 sweet mangoes, peeled, flesh chopped

2 bananas, chopped

1/2 cup almond milk (or low-fat milk)

5 ice cubes

Method

Place mango flesh in blender. Add bananas, milk and ice cubes. Blend until smooth. Serve immediately.

MANGO ICED TEA

Serves: 4
Preparation time: 10 minutes

Ingredients

2 ripe mangoes, skinned and chopped
2 black tea bags or 1 tbsp tea leaves
4 cups cold water
1/2 tbsp lime juice (or lemon juice)
raw sugar to sweeten
mint leaves for garnish

Method

Place tea bags in a teapot and add boiling water. Brew
for 5 minutes. Place tea in fridge. Place mango flesh in
a blender. Puree until smooth. Set aside. When tea is
cool, pour into a blender. Add mango puree and lime
juice and sugar. Blend until smooth. Serve in glasses
with ice cubes and garnished with a sprig of mint.

WATERMELON JUICE WITH MINT

Serves: 4 - 6

Preparation time: 10 minutes

Ingredients

1 watermelon, peeled, deseeded and chopped

2 tbsp fresh mint leaves, stalks removed, washed

6 ice cubes

Method

Place watermelon in blender with mint leaves and ice cubes. Blend. Pour into glasses and garnish with mint sprigs.

STRAWBERRY ALMOND MILKSHAKE

Serves: 4

Preparation time: 10 minutes

Ingredients

250g strawberries, fresh or frozen

2 1/2 cups almond milk

1/2 tsp pure vanilla extract

raw sugar for taste

2 scoops vanilla ice-cream (optional)

4 ice cubes

Method

Place ingredients in blender and blend well. Pour into glasses. Add a small scoop of vanilla ice-cream. Garnish with fresh strawberries.

MOSAMBI LIME JUICE

Serves: 2
Preparation time: 10 minutes

Ingredients

6 sweet limes, peeled and chopped
sugar or honey to taste

Method

Remove seeds from the limes. Place in blender. Strain
pulp through fine sieve. Discard pulp. Add sugar or
honey to the juice. Add ice cubes. Serve chilled.

THE INDIAN KITCHEN

HOW TO MAKE FRESH PANEER

You can use purchased cottage cheese to replace paneer in recipes or make paneer at home using the following easy recipe.

Ingredients

1 liter warm full cream milk

2 tbsp lemon juice

Method

Warm milk. Add lemon juice. Stir. Milk will curdle. Place milk in a piece of clean muslin and hang up with a bowl under it. Let the water drip. Then press paneer under a heavy weight. After 1 hour remove the weight and place on a cutting board. Cut into squares and keep covered in fridge.

HOW TO MAKE COCONUT MILK

Coconut milk can be purchased in cartons or tins and kept in the fridge. If fresh coconuts are available, you can make coconut milk using the following recipe.

Ingredients

1 fresh coconut, grated

Method

Grate coconut. Strain and press through a fine sieve. This liquid makes thick coconut milk. Set this aside. Then add a little warm water to the coconut flesh and place in a blender. Pulse on low and then blend. Strain through a sieve to make thin coconut milk. Both thick milk and thin milk can be stored in the fridge and used in Indian recipes.

HOW TO MAKE ALMOND MILK

Serves: 4 – 6
Preparation time: 30 minutes

Ingredients

1 cup blanched almonds
4 cups cold water

Method

Place almonds and water in blender. Pulse first and blend well. Strain twice through a sieve. Store in a covered container in the fridge. Use within 4 days of making.

HOW TO MAKE DRY CHAI SPICE MIX FOR TEA

Makes: One jar
Preparation time: 5 minutes

Ingredients

1 whole nutmeg

1g cloves

1/4 cup ginger powder

3 cm cinnamon stick

10g cardamom

2 tbsp fennel seeds

1/2 tsp black pepper

1/4 cup chopped lemon grass (optional)

1/4 cup dry rose petals (optional)

Method

Blend the ginger, nutmeg and cardamom together in a blender or food processor. Add the rest of the spices together. Store in airtight container in the fridge. Use to make an Indian chai tea.

HOW TO MAKE CHAI TEA

Method

Add 3/4 to 1 tsp of your chai spice mix to a small saucepan. Add water. Bring slowly to a boil. Remove pan from heat. Stand for 4 minutes. Add milk and sugar to pan. Bring to boil. Remove from heat. Add 2 tsp black tea leaves. Let brew for 3 minutes. Stir. Strain chai into a warm teapot. Pour into cups.

HOW TO MAKE PLAIN CHAPATTI

Makes: 10
Cooking time: 30 minutes

Ingredients

1 cup fine plain flour
1 cup whole meal flour, sieved
1/2 tsp salt

2 tbsp sunflower oil
3/4 cup warm water, as needed

Method

Place flours and salt on a bench. Add oil into the middle of the flour. Add water to make a soft, elastic dough. Knead dough until smooth. Break off small pieces. Roll each piece into a ball. Leave to rest for 10 minutes. Heat a lightly greased griddle until hot. Or you can use a fry pan, gas flame or barbecue griddle to cook. Using a rolling pin, roll out the dough balls to make thin tortilla shapes. Pick up each round and "clap" between hands in a circular motion to get rid of excess flour and prevent burning. When the griddle starts to smoke, place a chapatti on the griddle to cook. Use long handled metal tongs to turn, as soon as the chapatti bubbles up, about 30 seconds, flip over to the other side. Then take off the griddle and hold over a flame until the bread gets some brown spots and is puffed up (for an authentic look). Remove from flame. Place in a bread serving basket while you make the rest of the batch.

HOW TO MAKE PLAIN RICE

Serves: 4

Ingredients:

1 cup basmati rice

2 cups water

1 tsp sunflower oil

Method:

Wash rice and soak rice 15 minutes before cooking. Drain rice in a sieve. Place rice in a large saucepan. Add water with 1 tsp of oil (or butter) and bring slowly to the boil. Turn heat down to low. Cover saucepan with a tight fitting lid. Cook 15 minutes on low heat. Remove saucepan from heat. If rice is cooked but still appears wet, leave rice to stand in pan with lid on. Fluff up rice with a fork before serving.

HOW TO MAKE LEMON RICE

Serves: 4

Cooking time: 20 minutes

Ingredients

1 cup basmati rice, washed and drained

1 small lemon, washed, zested and juiced

1/4 tsp mustard seeds

3 green cardamom pods, crushed

sunflower oil

Method

Heat 1 tsp of sunflower oil. Cut the lemon zest into strips. Cook with spices until fragrant. Add rice. Add 2 cups of water. Bring to simmer on low heat. Cover pan with lid. Cook on low heat until water is absorbed. Fluff with a fork and add 1/4 tsp of lemon juice or more to taste. Serve hot.

HOW TO MAKE ZEERA RICE

Serves: 4

Cooking time: 30 minutes

Ingredients

1 cup basmati rice

3 cups water

2 tsp sunflower oil

1 large onion, peeled, finely chopped

2 tsp cumin seeds

1/2 cup water

coriander leaves, chopped (garnish)

Method

Wash rice and drain. Add rice into a large saucepan.
Add 3 cups of cold water. Bring to boil. Boil on low
heat until almost cooked. Remove from heat. Drain
rice. Heat 1 tbsp oil in a frying pan. Add onions. Fry
until golden brown taking care not to burn. Add cumin
seeds. Stir. Add rice and stir. Add 1/2 cup water. Cover
pan. Simmer until rice is absorbed. Remove from heat.
Let rice stand for 4 minutes. Serve hot. Garnish with
coriander leaves.

HEALTH BENEFITS OF SPICES, HERBS AND OTHER INGREDIENTS

You'll find ingredients, herbs and spices listed below. All with their key nutrients and healing properties. The herbs and spices have descriptions of minerals, vitamins, phytochemicals, folate and fiber properties. Phytochemicals contain antioxidants and enzyme-activating sulfur compounds. Enzyme-activating sulfur compounds help stimulate enzyme production that in turn help eliminate carcinogens. Antioxidants prevent chemical reactions called oxidation, which cause cancer.

Anise

Healing properties: Anise has been traditionally used to treat digestive and bronchial problems.

Key nutrient properties: Calcium, iron, manganese, potassium, zinc. Vitamin C, B6, B1, B3, A, E, folate, fiber. Phytochemicals.

Bay Leaves

Healing properties: Bay is used for relieving migraines. Also beneficial for the stomach and intestinal tract as bay leaf oil is antibacterial.

Key nutrient properties: Calcium, iron, manganese, potassium, zinc. Vitamin C, A, E, B2 (riboflavin) B3 (niacin) and folate. Phytochemicals.

Black Pepper

Healing properties: Aids digestion, natural antibiotic, relieves coughs and colds, clears congestion, fights cancer. Promotes absorption of nutrients - improving overall health. Increase the body's ability to absorb vitamins, minerals and proteins. Boosts metabolism and helps break down fat cells. Improves skin complexion.

Key nutrient properties: manganese, vitamin K, C, E, B2 (riboflavin) magnesium, iron, copper, fiber and phosphorus.

Cardamom

Healing properties: Cardamom is a member of the ginger family and like ginger is good for digestive system and helps relieve bronchitis and asthma. Stimulates appetite. Flushes toxins from the body. Increases blood circulation. Anti bacterial, anti fungal, anti carcinogenic.

Key nutrient properties: An outstanding source of manganese. I tsp has 26% of daily value. Calcium, iron, manganese, potassium, zinc. Vitamin C, A, E, B2 (riboflavin) B3 (niacin) and folate. Phytochemicals.

Cinnamon

Healing properties: Cinnamon helps relieve nausea, vomiting, diarrhea and indigestion. It has anti cancer properties and laboratory tests have shown it stops the growth of liver cancer and melanoma cells. Helps with type-2 diabetes because it lowers blood sugar levels and increase insulin production. Anti-fungal. Fights Candida. Boosts brain function and memory. Fights bad breath. A natural painkiller and potent antioxident.
Key nutrient properties: Calcium, iron, manganese, potassium, zinc, phosphorous. Vitamin C, B1, B2, B3, B6, folate and fiber. Phytochemicals.

Cloves
Healing properties: Cloves are used to aid digestion, kill intestinal parasites, help abdominal pain and symptoms of peptic ulcers. Boosts metabolism. Removes toxins from bloodstream. Contains blood purifying properties which support a healthy immune system. Improves cardiovasular health by preventing blood clots and regulating blood sugar levels. Higher than any food in antioxident content.
Key nutrient properties: Calcium, iron, manganese, potassium, zinc, phosphorous. Vitamin C, B2, B3, B6, folate and fiber. Phytochemicals.

Coriander
Healing properties: helps indigestion and diarrhea.
Key nutrient properties: Calcium, iron, manganese, potassium, zinc, phosphorous. Vitamin C, B1 (thiamine) B2 (riboflavin) B3 (niacin) B6, vitamin A, E (in leaf only) folate and fiber. Phytochemicals.

Cumin
Healing properties: Cumin is used for treating colic, headaches and aids digestion.
Key nutrient properties: Calcium, iron, manganese, potassium, zinc, phosphorous. Vitamin C, B1(thiamine), B2 (riboflavin) B3 (niacin) B6, vitamin A, E (in leaf only) folate and fiber. Phyto-

chemicals.

Fennel

Healing properties: Fennel aids kidney and bladder function. It's used for relieving nausea and motion sickness.
Key nutrient properties: Calcium, iron, manganese, potassium, zinc, phosphorous. Vitamin C, vitamin A, B1 (thiamine) B2 (riboflavin) B3 (niacin) fiber and folate. Phytochemicals.

Garlic

Garlic is well known for all its beneficial properties, but I am interested in its immune system supporting properties. Eating just one clove of garlic a day can help decrease cholesterol levels. Enzymes in garlic help in the synthesis of cholesterol.

Ginger

Healing properties: One of the most widely used medicinal herbs on earth. Traditional remedy for nausea, aids digestion, may help destroy Salmonella which causes food poisoning. It also known to destroy parasites and their eggs.
Helps with sore throats and destroys cold viruses.
Key nutrient properties: Calcium, iron, manganese, potassium, zinc, phosphorous. Vitamin C, vitamin A, vitamin E, B1 (thiamine) B2 (riboflavin) B3 (niacin) fiber and folate. Phytochemicals.

Mint

Healing properties: Eases insomnia, nervous tension and upset stomachs. Mint also increases the number of phagocytes which destroy bacteria, cancer cells and pathogens.
Key nutrient properties: Calcium, iron, manganese, potassium, zinc, phosphorous. Vitamin C, vitamin A, vitamin E, B1 (thiamine), B2 (riboflavin) B3 (niacin) B6, fiber and folate. Phytochemicals.

Mustard Seed

Healing properties: Loosens mucus and stimulates bronchial gland secretion. Helps nervous system function and regulates metabolism. Helps lower blood cholesterol. Protects the cells from harmful oxygen free radicals. Helps formation of red blood cells and cellular metabolism.

Key nutrient properties: Copper, calcium, sodium, selenium, iron, manganese, potassium, zinc, phosphorous. Vitamin C, vitamin A, vitamin E, B1 (thiamine), B2 (riboflavin), B3 (niacin), B6, fiber and folate. Phytochemicals.

Nutmeg

Healing properties: Nutmeg has antiviral and anti inflammatory properties. Eases vomiting, nausea and diarrhea.

Key nutrient properties: Copper, calcium, sodium, selenium, iron, manganese, potassium, zinc, phosphorous. Vitamin C, vitamin A, vitamin E, B6, fiber and folate. Phytochemicals.

Saffron

Healing properties: Saffron acts as an antioxidant and as a stimulant to the blood circulatory system.

Key nutrient properties: Calcium, sodium, selenium, iron, manganese, magnesium, potassium, zinc, phosphorous. Vitamin C, vitamin A, vitamin E, B1 (thiamine) B2 (riboflavin) B3 (niacin) B6, fiber and folate. Phytochemicals.

Turmeric

Healing properties: Improves blood vessel health, reduces cholesterol and is an important anti inflammatory herb in Ayurvedic medicine. Turmeric has also been shown to inhibit cancer.

Key nutrient properties: Calcium, selenium, iron, manganese, magnesium, potassium, zinc, phosphorous. Vitamin C, vitamin A, vitamin E, B1 (thiamine), B2 (riboflavin), B3 (niacin), B6, fiber and folate. Phytochemicals.

Fenugreek

Healing properties: Good laxative properties, reduces fever and helps lung disorders.

Key nutrient properties: Vitamins B1, B2, B3, B6, B12 and vitamin D. Folic acid, essential oils, iron and biotin.

Mustard (seeds)
Healing properties: Improves digestion and helps metabolize fat.

Rose
Healing properties: Good for infections and bladder issues. Also good for diarrhea.
Key nutrient properties: Vitamins A, B3, C, D, Zinc, flavonoids, fructose and sucrose.

Yogurt and Paneer
In his book *Diet and Diet Reform*, Mahatma Gandhi recommended yogurt as a staple to his people. Yogurt is an animal derived complete protein source. In Indian cooking yogurt and paneer (a cow based cottage style cheese) is used frequently in recipes, with good reason. Teeming with friendly bacteria, yogurt is milk thickened by good bacteria, Lactobacillus acidophilus, growing in it. More digestible than liquid cows' milk, yogurt is a great source of protein, calcium, potassium, vitamin B6, vitamin B12, vitamin B3 and folic acid. Yogurt is known to lower cholesterol levels, help in the fight against certain cancers, reduce the chance of strokes and heart attacks. The active "good" bacteria helps prevent and fight digestive tract infections, fight cholera, dysentery, diarrhea, aid digestion and food absorption, prevent bloating and help prevent some food allergies.

Mushrooms
Healing properties: Mushrooms help prevent heart disease. Boost the immune system. Protect the body from various cancer cells. High in copper which helps produce blood cells and maintain heart health.
Key nutrient properties: Contain protein, carbohydrates, fiber, vitamin C, vitamin E, calcium, iron, selenium, zinc and potassium.

Tomatoes
Healing properties: Tomatoes help the body resist infection and fight cancer. Potent anti cancer properties are not found in raw

tomatoes. Cooking releases Lycopene, the beneficial amino acid. Tomatoes can lower blood pressure, protect against digestive problems, help in cleansing toxins from the body and benefit the kidneys.

Plant/vegetable oils

Sunflower oil is used to cook many of the recipes in this book. Healing properties: Sunflower oil contains immune boosting vitamin E. Vegetable oils derived from plants, nuts and seeds are known to help reduce the risk of coronary artery disease.

Nuts

Many of the recipes call for cashew nuts, almonds and other nuts and seeds. Nuts, especially unsalted peanuts, cashews and almonds are high in monosaturated fats and are known to help lower cholesterol as well. As with all nuts in the recipes, make sure you use raw unsalted nuts.

Almonds

Healing properties: Known as the king of nuts. They are higher in fiber and calcium than any other nut. Good for the skin and highly nutritious. Rich in calcium, potassium, magnesium, phosphorous, folic acid, B vitamins, vitamin E and protein.

Cashews

Healing properties: Primarily grown in India and used extensively in Indian recipes for main dishes, breads, vegetables and desserts. High in protein, fiber, calcium, iron, potassium, magnesium, vitamin A, zinc, B vitamin and vitamin E. They contain essential amino acids and are high in monounsaturated fatty acids, good for the heart and circulation.

Pistachio nuts

Healing properties: Pistachios are one of the highest sources of potassium of all the nuts. With a sweet flavor, they make great snacks and desserts. Pistachios are high in protein, fiber, calcium, iron, magnesium, phosphorous, potassium, zinc, manganese, vitamin C, vitamin B's, folate and vitamins E and A.

Melon Seeds
Healing properties: High in vitamin B, essential fatty acids, protein and zinc. Good for skin disorders.

Coconut
Healing properties: One cup of coconut milk contains 89mg of magnesium. This helps the nervous system. Packed with vitamin C, E, B1, B3, B5, B6, iron, selenium, calcium, magnesium and phosphorous. Coconut gives a boost of energy as it has electrolytes. Fifty percent of the fatty acid in coconut oil is lauric acid which fights a variety of microrganisms, including, yeast, bacteria, fungi and viruses. High in manganese which helps metabolize glucose and regulate blood sugar levels.

Lemons and limes
Healing properties: Citrus fruits help lower cholesterol and stops cholesterol from forming plaques in the arteries.

Basmati rice
Healing properties: Rich in complex carbohydrates, yet low in fat and calories. Contains protein and high levels of lysine, an amino acid. Rice helps digestion and helps the body recover in acute bouts of diarrhea. It helps regulate glucose metabolism in people with diabetes.

MENIERE MAN BOOKS

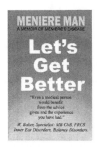

Let's Get Better
A Memoir of Meniere's Disease

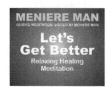

Let's Get Better CD
Relaxing & Healing Guided Meditation Voiced by Meniere Man

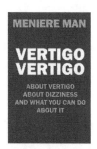

Vertigo Vertigo
About Vertigo About Dizziness and What You Can Do About it.

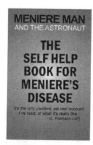

Meniere Man And The Astronaut
The Self Help Book for Meniere's Disease

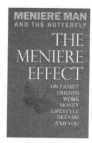

Meniere Man And The Butterfly The Meniere Effect
How to Minimize the Effect of Meniere's on Family, Money, Lifestyle, Dreams and You.

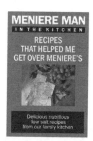

Meniere Man In The Kitchen. Recipes That Helped Me Get Over Meniere's
Delicious nutritious low salt recipes from our family kitchen.

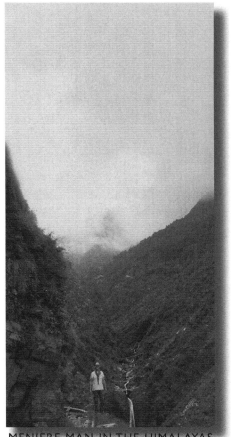

MENIERE MAN IN THE HIMALAYAS

ABOUT THE AUTHOR

At the height of his business career and aged just forty-six, he suddenly became acutely ill. He was diagnosed with Meniere's disease, but the full impact of having Meniere's disease was to come later. He was to lose not only his health, but his career and financial status as well. He also began to lose all hope that he would fully recover a sense of well-being.

It was his personal spirit and desire to get "back to normal" that changed his life for the better. He decided that you can't put a limit on anything in life. Rather than letting Meniere's disease get in the way of recovery, he started to focus on what to do about getting over Meniere's disease. And that's just what he went on to do.

These days life is different for the Author. He is a fit active man who has no symptoms of Meniere's disease except for hearing loss and tinnitus in one ear. Following his own advice he continues to avoid salt, stress, takes vitamins, exercises regularly and maintains a positive, mindful attitude. He does not take any medication.

All the physical activities he enjoys these days require a high degree of balance and equilibrium: snowboarding, surfing, hiking, windsurfing, weightlifting, and riding a motorbike, (activities he started to do while suffering with Meniere's disease).

He writes books on Meniere's in the hope that his experience and management techniques will help others find a way to manage symptoms and ultimately get over Meniere's disease. He has a firm belief that if you want to experience a marked improvement in health, you can't wait until you feel well to start. You must begin to improve your health now, even though you may not feel like it. The more you do, the more you can do.

Today the Author is a writer, painter, designer and exhibiting artist. He is married to a Poet. They have two adult children. He spends most days writing or painting. He enjoys the sea, cooking, travel, photography, nature and the great company of family, friends and his beloved dog.

MENIERE SUPPORT NETWORKS

Meniere's Society (UNITED KINGDOM)
www. menieres.org.uk
Meniere's Society Australia (AUSTRALIA)
info@menieres.org.au
The Meniere's Resource & Information Centre (AUSTRALIA) www.
menieres.org.au
Healthy Hearing & Balance Care (AUSTRALIA)
www.healthyhearing.com.au
Vestibular Disorders association (AUSTRALIA)
www.vestibular .org
The Dizziness and Balance Disorders Centre (AUSTRALIA)
www.dizzinessbalancedisorders.com
Meniere's Research Fund Inc   (AUSTRALIA)
www.menieresresearch.org.au
Australian Psychological Society APS (AUSTRALIA)
www.psychology.org.au
Meniere's Disease Information Center (USA)
www.menieresinfo.com
Vestibular Disorders Association (USA)
www.vestibular.org
BC Balance and Dizziness Disorders Society (CANADA)
www.balanceand dizziness.org
WebMD.
www.webmd.com
National Institute for Health
www.medlineplus.gov
Mindful Living Program
www.mindfullivingprograms.com
Center for Mindfulness
www. umassmed.edu.com

FACEBOOK SITES
Meniere Resources Inc
The Meniere's Society
Living with Meniere's
Meniere's Australia
Seattle Dizzy Group
Meniere Disease Awareness
Balancing Meniere's

Made in the USA
San Bernardino, CA
15 March 2015